THE

GENTLEMAN'S HAND-BOOK

OF

HOMŒOPATHY;

ESPECIALLY FOR TRAVELERS,

AND FOR

DOMESTIC PRACTICE.

BY

EGBERT GUERNSEY, M.D.

AUTHOR OF "DOMESTIC PRACTICE."

BOSTON:
PUBLISHED BY OTIS CLAPP, 3 BEACON ST.
NEW YORK·
WILLIAM RADDE, 322 BROADWAY.
1855.

W. H. TINSON, Stereotyper,
24 Beekman St., N. Y.

PREFACE.

Freedom of thought, and a love of scientific investigation, are prominent characteristics of the present generation. In every branch of society, in every department of life, the mists of error, prejudice, and ignorance, are rapidly fading away. The cry is now everywhere, "What is truth?" and shadowy forms, and fine-drawn theories, are giving place to the real and substantial, the positive revelations of science. These revelations are not now confined to a favored few, but are broadly disseminated and eagerly received among all classes of community. Nowhere is this more true than with that science whose investigations are directed to the relief of human suffering.

This freedom of inquiry among the masses stimulates the profession and urges them on to careful and candid investigation. The more the people understand the laws of their being, the better will they be enabled to prevent disease, and the more careful and thorough will the profession become.

Strong objections have been made against works of Domestic Practice, on the ground that familiarity with the symptoms of disease may so work on the imagination as to produce disease, and also from the great danger of laymen attempting to meddle with drugs.

The first objection is too puerile to deserve notice, and the second would have more force when applied to a school whose gentlest weapons are lancets and cathartics.

Neither objection would have weight in a work of this kind. It is not intended to make every man his own physician; but there are times and places where a physician cannot be obtained, and when immediate aid is necessary. There are other cases perfectly plain and simple, where an ordinary capacity can apply the remedy with an assurance of success.

Designing this work especially for gentlemen, it has been our object to make plain those laws of their being which will enable them to ward off disease, and shunning vice and its fearful consequences, harmonize their passions, and make them not alone healthier, but better. Believing much of the disease in the world is the result of improper marriages, we have introduced some important facts upon that subject. We have also directed the attention to different mineral springs, changes of climate, and directions for travelers. In the part on the treatment of disease, we have been as plain, simple, and concise as possible, speaking more particularly of the more common class of diseases. It is in the early stage of some simple trouble, such as cold or dyspepsia, that the seeds are planted of the worst and most torturing forms of disease. Meeting these symptoms at the commencement with a few easily chosen remedies, long attacks of suffering may be prevented, and even life itself saved. Toward the close of the work, chapters have been introduced on injuries occasioned by accidents, apparent death, poisons, and their antidotes, and electricity.

Every effort has been made to make this work as plain, practical, and concise as possible.

NEW YORK, 1855,
19 West 22d St.

CONTENTS.

CHAPTER I.

CHAPTER II.

CHAPTER III.

CHAPTER IV.

PART II.

CHAPTER I.

CHAPTER II.

CHAPTER III.

CHAPTER IV.

CHAPTER V.

CHAPTER VI.

CHAPTER X.

CHAPTER XI.

CHAPTER XII.

CHAPTER XIII.

CHAPTER XIV.

GENTLEMAN'S HAND-BOOK

OF

HOMŒOPATHY.

CHAPTER I.

HUMAN LIFE.

It is a mournful sight to look out upon the heaving ocean, when the sky is dark with storm, and see the proud ship, freighted with wealth and human life, struggling fearfully, yet vainly, to avoid impending destruction, go down in the boiling waters.

How much more sad to gaze upon the wrecks which strew so thickly the vast ocean of life; human wrecks, in comparison with which the proud ship, a shattered navy, or the temples and half buried cities of a past age crumbling before the march of time, sink into insignificance.

Men go about with bent forms, and bowed down heads, with disease and death stamped upon their faces ere they have reached man's estate, or rush along life's pathway with eager haste and flashing eye, heedless of danger, reckless of life.

No wonder that the grave closes over them in early prime ; no wonder that their shrieks pierce the air, from the maniac cell, or that the wrecks of men, sad and wasted, going down to death, are scattered all along the journey of life.

But the fault has not commenced with this generation. Men have not grown suddenly reckless of life, have not become in one generation the puny, sickly race we see, some of them with bodies too strong for the mind, wearing it out in their headlong speed, and others with mind and body both sickly and debased. No ; we are hurried along on the swift current of a stream whose source is in the darkness of the past. Here and there the waters emerge from the darkness and flash clear and sparkling in the bright sunlight. Greece, worshipping beauty, sculptures it in matchless forms of art, blends it in palace and temple, and wakens the echoes of coming ages with the matchless songs of Homer. Plato discourses of immortality from the groves of the academy, and the stern patriot falters not at duty even though it desolates his own home

Rome, treading for awhile the conquerer's path, making its literature the world's classic, at length bends the knee to barbarian hosts. But Greece and Rome contained within themselves seeds of dissolution, in the moral depravity, which tainted as with a leper's touch every class of society. The palaces of their emperors and the temples of their gods, became but little more than brothels, within which were practiced the most hellish forms of pollution. Then followed the age of physical force. The ponderous sword, the mighty battle-ax, wielded by sinewy arms, the hand-to-hand fight, were the playthings and pleasures of life. Men, as it regards physical strength, towered up like giants, strong and vigorous. But still in their midst vice lifted its head, and with each succeeding generation scattered its seeds more broadly over the world. Then came the whirlwind march of Revolution, dashing thrones to earth, and shaking the world like the throes of an earthquake.

Oh, what a sad picture does the world present for the past six thousand years. History itself is but little more than a record, with a few bright exceptions, of wrong, and crime, and dark depravity ; the strong trampling upon the weak, and the vile tainting the pure and holy : almost every page is written with blood and stained with tears wrung from suffering hearts.

As man was created, how noble and God-like he stands forth, the most sublime and glorious of all his Creator's works. As the current of his life has flowed on through the corruption of past ages, how like a pigmy he seems, with his weakened body, his groaning and sighing, his petty ambition and narrow and selfish ends and aims. The politician, struggling for the spoils and honors of office ; the eager crowd jostling along life's pathway in pursuit of wealth, which when acquired they know not how to enjoy, drones of society, vegetating through life, living on the fruits of their fathers' toil, devotees to fashion and slaves to sensual passions. The man of business throws himself heart and soul into the pursuit of gain; the student toils on over the midnight lamp, heedless of the hectic flush and the wasting frame; the young man stepping out upon the theatre of action, giddy with the whirl and roar of life around him, is apt to rush from the toils of business into the various avenues of vice which open so thickly around him; and all forget one great truth, the intimate relation existing between body and mind, and unless both are kept active, pure and healthy, every organ performing its specific duty, withering disease, a soul tossed by the whirlwind of passion, or fretted and unhappy, will be the inevitable result.

Borne along by the rushing tide which surges and dashes around us, we do not pause to think, but yield to the impulses and passions which a corrupt and unhealthy society has fastened upon us, disregard the laws of physical health, and rush madly into the jaws of danger and death.

Oh, how thickly the earth is piled with graves of the young! how it groans beneath its load of human suffering, oppression and wrong! And is all this right? Are these pigmy forms, wasted by disease, or deformed by passion, the men God made in his own image and placed in a world of beauty?

Look abroad upon nature, and one great law pervades all—harmony and beauty. See it in shining worlds, sweeping in circles of light around their great parent center ; hear it in the song of the bird as it cleaves the air, filling it with wild notes of melody ; see it in forest tree and lowly flower, in the gorgeous tints of autumn—the hectic flush of a dying year—and the opening, budding beauties of spring.

Look now upon Man, that crowning glory of God's works, and where is the beauty and harmony of purity and truth?

Listen to the wail of the dying from the gory battle-field, to the groans of the oppressed, to the pulsations of that heart whose every throb is narrow selfishness, to the midnight revel, to the discord and jar of life—sum up the mighty record of diseases which devastate the world, and then may we not well say, "How has God's most noble work become involved in ruin! how have the mighty fallen, and the most fine gold become dim!"

Surrounded as we are by temptations, with the current of our life tainted by flowing on through the corrupt generations of the past, with the seeds of death rankling within us, and disease and death meeting us at every step, may we not, by adhering closely to nature's laws, cleanse that tainted current, pluck out some, at least, of those seeds of early death, and harmonize our passions, so that the vile and flaunting weeds which have taken such deep root within us may wither, and the germs of the holy, the beautiful and the true, grow up and expand in fragrant loveliness. Then will the great human heart pulsate in unison with the Divine; then will earth, renewing its youth, bear upon its smiling bosom an emancipated race.

Were we living in a state of Eden purity, the instincts of our nature might, if we gave heed to them, protect us from harm, and like the birds, need trouble ourselves no more than they about the mechanism of our being and the laws of nature. But we must not forget that for ages on ages, violation of nature's laws has tainted life's current with disease, and that we have within us impurities which, unless we walk with cautious footsteps, will develop themselves in a ripe harvest of suffering. It is well for us to ascertain, then, the necessities of our being and the laws of life.

CHAPTER II.

PHYSIOLOGY AND HYGIENE.

WITHIN the human system we have the most perfect chemical laboratory ever constructed. From the food we eat, the water we drink, and the air we breathe, it prepares for the bones the materials necessary for their growth and waste ; sends to the muscles, the eyes, the teeth, the brain and the nerves, each the component parts required for their life and the performance of their duties, and develops in its varied combinations the animal heat which keeps up the equilibrium of life.

The first step which the food undergoes in this chemical change, is in the mouth. Here ground and triturated by the action of the teeth, and thoroughly mixed with the salivary juice, it is prepared for the stomach. But this step, apparently so simple, is of the utmost importance. The salivary juice aids materially the process of digestion, and unless the food is slowly and thoroughly masticated the glands remain partially inactive and the saliva is only mixed to a small extent with the food. The stomach, therefore, suffers by being compelled to receive food not prepared for its use. It suffers also from the habit, by far too common, of washing down the food with copious draughts of water, coffee, or tea. But very little liquid should be taken at meals, for it not only checks the salivary secretion, but by diluting the gastric juice weakens the action of the stomach. Very hot food or drink stimulates to an undue degree, for a certain time, the vessels of the mouth and stomach, to be followed in a short time by reaction, loss of tone and strength. Decayed teeth, spongy gums, and indigestion, are the results.

Time of Eating.—The food should be taken at regular intervals, so as to give the stomach ample time, not only to thoroughly digest and empty its contents, but to rest and rally its powers before the next meal. The habit so peculiarly American, of rushing through the meal in hot haste, as if life itself depended on the rapidity with which the food was bolted, and among business men and students in particular, of eating at all hours, catching it whenever and wherever they can get it, is the fruitful cause of torturing attacks of indigestion, fretfulness, and peevishness of disposition, headache, palpitation of the heart, constipation, hypochondria, and a host of ailments. The complaints of the stomach are immediately telegraphed through the pneumogastric nerve to the brain, and from thence through the nervous system to every part of the body; so that the whole system is likely to suffer from the derangement of this organ, and the diseases thus engendered sometimes break down the constitution and terminate life. Cancerous and tubercular diseases are sometimes produced by long-continued indigestion.

Kind and Quantity of Food.—The kind and quantity of food should be governed, in a great measure, by climate, constitution and habits of life. Experience teaches us that the inhabitants of warm climates do not require as much strong food as those of colder regions, nor persons of sedentary life as much as those engaged in active pursuits.

Food is the fuel, which develops in its combustion the animal heat, which warms us in cold and keeps up the even temperature of the blood, in all climates, and under every external circumstance. Experiment has shown that the temperature of the blood in health, in summer and winter, in the heat of the tropics and the intense cold of the frigid regions, is nearly the same.

This will not appear strange when we look upon the animal body as a heated mass, giving out heat when the surrounding objects are cooler than itself, and taking it in when they are warmer.

What an enormous difference there must be in the

amount of heat given out in these warm climates where the temperature is nearly the same as the body, and in those intensely cold regions where it is 100° lower, and what a vast difference there must also be in the amount of food required to keep up that combustion, which produces animal heat.

Deprive the native of the South of food, and death would be slow in its progress, while the inhabitant of a frozen region, deprived of food, would speedily die. In the latter case, the enormous combustion required to be kept up to defend the system against cold, would in a short time exhaust the body of its carbon, and death would ensue.

Satisfactory experiments show that an adult, performing moderate exercise in a temperate climate, takes into the system through the lungs, from the atmospheric air, a little over thirty-two ounces of oxygen daily, and consumes in the form of food thirteen or fourteen ounces of carbon per day. This oxygen uniting with the carbon, forms carbonic acid, a portion of which is thrown off from the lungs ; another portion uniting with the hydrogen, forms the perspiration and urine, which pass off through the skin and kidneys. The result of this union is the combustion which produces animal heat.

Food Governed by Climate and Habits of Life.—It is evident, then, that the amount of carbon consumed in the healthy system must be in proportion to the oxygen taken into the body. The amount of oxygen inspired depends upon the frequency of the respirations and the temperature of climate. In warm climates the air is not only highly rarefied, but contains a considerable amount of water, so that but little oxygen is introduced, and comparatively a small amount of carbon is required in the food. Nature has kindly provided for this, for the fruits and vegetables which compose a large portion of the food of the natives of tropical climates, contain but about twelve per cent. of carbon, while the meat and train oil which are so freely eaten in frigid regions, contain about eighty per cent.

In warm climates, then, the food should be light, consisting principally of fruits and vegetables, and that class of food which contains but little fat, and therefore requires but little oxygen for its combustion. If the stomach is crowded with meats and food rich in carbon, the food is not consumed, but goes to form fat, or clogs up the system, renders the stomach and liver inactive, and develops those fevers which are so terrible to the unacclimated. The stomach must be kept active, for here the food, by means of the gastric juice, which is slightly acid, is prepared to enter into the circulation. The liver must also perform its duty, for through this the venous blood passes on its way to the heart, and its office is to take up those particles which in the combustion are not entirely consumed, and those chemical combinations which with a little change may again enter the circulation. The bile thus secreted by the liver is strongly alkaline, and being poured into the lower stomach neutralizes the acidity of the food now reduced to chyme, and renders it fit to be taken up by the absorbents which open with their little mouths upon the intestinal canal, taking up the nutriment and pouring it into the thoracic duct, from whence it is conveyed through the arterial system to every part of the body. If the stomach is inactive, the food is not digested, and if the liver is torpid, no bile is secreted from the blood, so that all the impurities which this organ should have taken up, sweep on through the system, irritating and inflaming the blood, and giving rise to serious forms of disease.

For the same reason that fruits, vegetables, and food, containing but little carbon—or fat—should be used in warm climates, strong nourishing food, such as meats and grains rich in carbon, should be eaten in cold climates. The more laborious exercise a person performs, and the more he is exposed to the inclemency of the weather, the stronger and more nourishing should be his food. The air in these cold regions is more condensed, so that at each inspiration a much larger amount of oxygen is inspired than in warmer climates, and the combustion is consequently much more rapid. This rapid development of animal heat is absolutely essential to guard against the cold, which, were it not for this internal fire, would rapidly prostrate the vital powers.

There are many tribes of Indians who go almost naked, but they consume a vast amount of carbon in the meat, train oil and tallow, which form their food. Clothes, after all, are only an equivalent for a certain amount of food.

The food then, both in kind and quantity, should conform to climate and occupation. In persons of sedentary life, the change of tissue is not as great, the circulation not so active, and therefore, on account of there being less waste in the system, the same amount of food, either in strength or quantity, is not required as in those of active life. If taken into the system it is not consumed and indigestion or obesity will probably be the result.

Varieties of Food.—A person should not sit down to a hearty meal immediately after taking violent exercise, for the system weakened by fatigue should have a few moments' time to rally; neither should he go directly from the table to his labor, but allow the stomach twenty or thirty minutes' time to direct its entire energies to the digestion of its contents. For a similar reason should a person abstain from food immediately before retiring to rest ; for the process of digestion is in a measure suspended during sleep, and the presence of food in the stomach at that time would be likely to cause a restless night and future trouble.

Ripe fruits are as a general thing perfectly harmless, both in sickness and health. It is better, however, to eat them in the early part of the day. In health the stomach should be sufficiently strong to digest proper food without the aid of stimulants either in cooking or in drinks. The more plain and simple the cooking the better.

Pork is difficult of digestion, and should never be used by persons of a scrofulous habit. Mutton, beef, vension and poultry, are not only highly nutritious but easy of digestion. Veal and lamb are nutritious, but not as easy of digestion. Eggs and milk are highly nutritious, but they sometimes produce headache and derangement of the stomach. Oysters are usually easy of digestion when not cooked hard. The most nutritious grains are wheat and Indian corn. Rice is nutritious and easy of digestion as well as sago, arrow root, tapioca, and farina.

THE NERVOUS SYSTEM.

The brain, the seat of the nervous system, is a soft, pulpy, grayish mass, occupying the cavity formed by the bones of the skull, and sending its influence through the nerves, to every part of the system.

The nerves usually pass off from the brain and spinal cord in pairs, one being the medium of sensation, and the other of motion. The one communicates feeling to and from the brain to every part of the body, and the other gives the power of motion to the muscular system.

Through these two-fold system of nerves, passing from the brain and communicating like a net-work with every part of the body, the functions of life are carried on, we move, breathe, eat and drink. Through the nerves, the eye takes in the glorious pictures of nature, the soul thrills to the touch of love, or vibrates to the harmony of music.

The brain, through the electric fluid generated in its batteries, sends its mandates along its telegraphic wires, the nerves, to the most remote part of the system, and the muscles hasten to obey. This sympathetic chain connects every part of the system with the great center, transmitting external sensations to the brain, and conveying the nervous fluid outward to the necessary place.

If, then, the nervous system performs such a prominent part in the economy of life, the necessity of keeping it vigorous, active, and healthy, and the danger of increasing or diminishing its sensibility by stimulants or narcotics, will be apparent.

The brain should not be overworked.—The records of disease show that insanity and affections of the heart have increased within the past few years to an alarming extent. In these feverish times, when fortunes are made or lost almost in a day, when to pause is to be borne down by the headlong crowd, rushing along the same path, and in pursuit of the same object, the mind is kept constantly on the stretch, and tasked to the utmost every day and every hour. The merchant marking out new fields of enterprise, and tasking the energies of his mind in perfecting and carrying out his plans, is liable, in his absorbing pursuits, to neglect those physical requirements essential to health. The mind must have rest as well as every other organ of the body, and when it is constantly tasked to the utmost, and never permitted to turn for recreation into other channels of thought, and especially when this is combined with a lack of care for physical health, the result is often incurable diseases of the heart, severe forms of nervous derangement, and insanity.

A great fault with those in active life, is, they live too fast, are too much immersed in the feverish whirl of business, and have but little time for healthy physical recreation, and the soothing charms of a happy home.

Derangement of the nervous system, occasioned either by disobedience of physical laws, by developing 'only one part of the mind, and one set of faculties or feelings, or by any other cause, shortens life, impairs usefulness, and embitters what might be our brimming cup of happiness. The more we live in obedience to the simple teachings of nature, the less likely shall we be to require artificial stimulants. When these stimulants are required, it shows conclusively that there is something wrong about the system.

Alcoholic drinks.—The effects of alcoholic drinks, when taken in large quantities, on the nervous system, are familiar to all. The trembling hand, the bowed and tottering form, the bloated face, and all the signs of premature old age, show their fearful ravages on the human system. The larger portion of the wine and brandy consumed, contain but a very small trace of the pure liquors whose names they bear. The drugs which enter into their composition, often produce on the system all the effects of slow poison. Reaction is sure to follow the excitement, both to the circulation and the nervous system, produced by the free use of alcoholic drinks, and the effects, slow at first, perhaps, in their progress, will sooner or later become apparent, in weakness of different organs, and deranged general health.

When stimulants in the form of alcoholic drinks are required, they should as a general thing be used by the advice of a judicious physician.

Tobacco.—The action of opium and tobacco on the nervous system, when freely used, is prejudicial to health.

The use of tobacco, when introduced into England by Sir Walter Raleigh, was very general throughout the western continent. It received in England but little favor at the hands of royalty. Elizabeth published an edict against its indulgence. James not only imposed severe pecuniary fines to abolish its use, but published his famous "Counterblaste to Tobacco," in which he remarks that smoking is a custom "loathsome to the eye, hateful to the nose, harmful to the brain, dangerous to the lungs; and in the black, stinking fume thereof, nearest resembling the horrible Stygian smoke of the pit that is bottomless."

In the sixteenth century, the king prohibited the use of tobacco in Persia; but as the punishment was penal, many of his subjects, rather than discontinue it, fled to the mountains. In 1624, Urban VIII. excommunicated all snuff-takers who committed the heinous sin of taking a pinch in church; and in the same century, the Russians, whose peasantry now smoke all day long, were forbidden to smoke under the penalty of having the nose cut off.

In Constantinople, where the use of tobacco in every form is now as common almost as eating, every Turk who was found smoking, was conducted in ridicule through the streets, with a pipe transfixed through his nose, and seated on an ass, with his face towards the tail; one reason was the supposition that the use of tobacco rendered the men impotent, and certainly, if taken in excess, such a result is likely to follow.

Notwithstanding all this opposition to tobacco, it still sent up its curling wreaths of defiance, until now it is used by every class of society the world over. When taken in sufficient quantity, it acts as a most virulent poison of the acro-narcotic class, producing deadly sickness, vertigo, and sometimes stupor. When tobacco is used in any shape to excess, it blunts the sensibility, not only of the organs with which it comes in contact, but of the whole nervous system; or it induces so great a susceptibility to impressions, that existence becomes painful. Snuffing is, perhaps, the least injurious mode of employing tobacco, yet even in this form, when used to excess, it is apt to induce dyspepsia, blunt the sensibility of the olfactory nerves, and change the tone of the voice, rendering it disagreeably nasal.

Tobacco contains two active principles, *nicotin* and a *volatile oil*. The former, acting through the pulmonary nerves, affects the circulation, and when the tobacco is used in large quantities, or in individuals unaccustomed to its use, may paralyze the heart.

In chewing, both the *nicotin* and *volatile oil* are

brought in contact with the mouth. Not only does it act injuriously upon the system in this way, but has a tendency to produce dyspepsia, by diverting from the food the gastric juice so useful in digestion.

In the moderate use of tobacco, the system may become habituated to its employment. When, however, indulgence becomes abuse, the nerves become unstrung; stupor, indisposition to mental or corporeal exertion, tremors, nausea, and the whole tribe of dyspeptic complaints supervene, and the victim finds his existence burdensome to himself as well as those around him.

Those, however, who persist in indulging in bad habits, should remember there is a time and place for everything. Either smoking or chewing, in the public street, is a disgusting habit, of which no gentleman should be guilty. The air of heaven belongs to all, and no one has a right to poison it by tainting it with the fumes of tobacco, or mark his passage through life by a stream of tobacco juice.

RESPIRATION AND CIRCULATION.

At each inspiration we take into the lungs about one pint of air. This, filling the air vessels, comes in contact with a surface which would cover more than twenty times the size of the human form. Separated from the air-cells by only a thin membrane are the blood vessels, filled with venous blood, which throw off, through this thin membrane, carbonic acid, and take in return oxygen from the air. The blood, having thus, by throwing off through the lungs a portion of its impurities, and receiving in the oxygen vitality from the air, changed its character to bright arterial blood, flows on to the heart, from which it is sent through the arterial system to every part of the body. When it has performed its life-giving functions, it passes on from the minute vessels which form the termination of the arteries, into the veins. These flowing into each other, carry the blood, now dark and venous, to the heart, from whence it passes to the lungs, there to be rendered fit to again pass through the system. Each cavity of the heart holds about two ounces, and as the heart contracts about seventy times in a minute, more than *two hogsheads* traverse it every hour. And yet, performing this mighty labor, it beats on, year after year, until paralyzed by death.

Necessity of Pure Air.—The necessity not only of having the lungs strong and fully developed, but the air taken into them pure and healthy, will be apparent to all. Impure air, poisoned with noxious exhalations from decaying animal and vegetable matter, brought in contact, not only with the immense surface of the air-vessels of the lungs, but with the entire circulation of the blood, diseases the lungs, and poisons the currents of life at their very fountain. The origin of pestilential diseases, which ravage cities, and carry death and weeping into almost every family, if it could be unfolded, would be found, in almost every instance, in some change of the atmospheric air.

That change, it is true, is sometimes beyond our control ; the air may be dry and hot, the heavens giving no rain, and the earth parched beneath our feet ; but the seeds of death too often fill the air from streets reeking with filth, from decaying animal and vegetable matter, which, with ordinary care, might have been removed, and take root, not only in systems impoverished from lack of proper healthy nourishment, but in the pampered sons and daughters of wealth, who, in the midst of luxury, daily violate nature's laws.

I need not speak of the necessity of well-ventilated rooms, both at home and in places of business, for the good sense of the age is now fairly aroused to the importance of pure air ; and, under the guiding hand of science, the time is not far distant when all buildings, designed to be occupied by human beings, will be constructed with an eye to comfort and health. Thanks, also, to the inventive spirit of our countrymen, the day is not far distant when we can travel by rail-car without fear of breathing air tainted by a hundred breaths, or of being choked by cinders and dust.

Development of the Chest.—The amount of oxygen introduced into the system must, of course, be guided in a measure by the size and strength of the lungs. The muscles of the chest then, by whose action respiration is carried on, should be strong and active, the chest well developed, and the respiration full and deep, filling the lungs with air Let man maintain, then, the erect form and noble bearing designed by nature. With chest broad and full, and head erect, there is something majestic in his appearance, something to inspire respect and confidence, while in the crouching form, the bent head, the narrow and contracted chest, there is, to say the least, an appearance of physical weakness and deformity.

Any position which has a tendency to throw the shoulders forward, contracts the chest, narrows the capacity of the lungs, interferes materially, not only with circulation, but digestion, and through them with the nutrition and health of the whole system. As exercise is essential to the growth of any organ, those whose employment is of a sedentary character, giving but little exercise to the chest, should resort to artificial means to keep it healthy and active. Fencing, and that class of amusements which brings into active play the arms, develops also the muscles of the chest. Vocal music, aside, when properly performed, of being a most valuable exercise to the voice and chest, is, also, a charming accomplishment, and an invaluable aid to the fascinations of social life.

FUNCTIONS OF THE SKIN.

The lungs, however well developed, strong, and active, cannot perform, with safety, more than their due proportion of labor. When we take into consideration that the body is a heated mass, within which combustion is constantly going on, and that, not only a vast amount of heat radiates from its surface, but, through the almost innumerable pores of the skin, perspiration is constantly passing off, charged with various chemical compounds, the result of the internal combustion and change of tissue all the time going on, we perceive the immense importance of keeping the skin healthy and active.

The structure of the skin shows in a strong light those wondrous marks of beauty and utility which meet us at every step in the investigation of the human system. To the naked eye, the skin is apparently composed of but one membrane ; yet, in reality, it consists of two. The outer layer is called the *cuticle* or *scarf skin,* is horny in its structure, insensible to pain, and guards the nervous, sensitive, *true skin,* or internal layer, from the constant pain it would experience from being brought in contact with material objects, and the harsh wind and dust.

The true skin is exceedingly sensitive, and contains, not only *arteries, veins* and *nerves,* but *oil glands* and *perspiratory glands.* The arteries and veins are very numerous, dividing and subdividing into innumerable capillary vessels, forming a beautiful vascular net-work. The nerves, which spread over every part of the sensitive layer of the true skin, proceed from the spiral cord, so that the brain is in direct communication with every part of the body ; for, not the point of a needle can penetrate the skin without reaching some one of these nervous filaments. Thus, by a wise provision of Providence, are we guarded from danger, for the sensation from external objects is immediately communicated to the brain.

The oil glands keep the skin soft and elastic by their oily secretions, and the perspiratory glands, through their little ducts, carry off an immense amount, in the form of perspiration of chemical compounds, the result of internal combustion and change of tissue, which would otherwise be thrown back upon internal organs, clogging them in their movements, producing fever and pain.

These little ducts or pores are about a quarter of an inch in length, and number about 7,000,000, so that in an ordinary sized person, the length of perspiratory tube is nearly *twenty-eight miles.* This immense apparatus for carrying off the waste of the system, in health, is in constant action. If, then, the external openings of these almost innumerable ducts are closed, either from lack of cleanliness, sudden change of temperature, or other cause, their work must be performed, if performed at all, by other organs—the liver, the lungs, bowels, or kidneys—resulting, not unfrequently, in serious disease of vital organs, and derangement of the entire system.

BATHING.

With these facts before us, we have some of the most powerful arguments, not only for cleanliness, but a proper external temperature of the body. The use of water may be either beneficial or injurious, according to the manner in which it is applied.

The application of a medium colder than the temperature of the body, produces a contraction of the capillary vessels, forcing the blood inward. The primary effect of cold bathing is sedative, but if the person is robust, and the power of generating heat active and vigorous, the internal heat soon forces the blood to the surface, and the first cold shivering sensation is speedily followed by a glow of warmth. It is in these cases that cold bathing is beneficial. Where the application of cold water is speedily followed, when friction is used, by a warm glow, and increased vigor and strength, no danger need be apprehended from its full use. The daily use of the sponge bath, in these cases, fortifies the system against cold, and renders the person less likely to suffer from change of temperature.

Persons of weakly constitution and sluggish circulation, with but slight power of generating animal heat, or persons of highly excitable nervous temperament or plethoric habits, cannot always bear cold bathing. Reaction, notwithstanding the most vigorous friction, is slow in taking place, lassitude and languor, or nervous derangement is the result. In these cases immersing the body in cold water should be avoided, and the tepid bath substituted. The cold sponge bath can be used by almost every one, as the shock is not great, and vigorous friction will, in almost every case, be followed in a few moments by warmth. In cold weather the room should be moderately warm. The tepid bath, to the feeble and enervated frame, is one of the greatest luxuries in the world. Its temperature should be guided by the feelings of the patient being sufficiently warm to produce no shock to the system. If higher than the temperature of the blood, or about 98°, it is followed by profuse perspiration, and the system is weakenod.

The temperature of the water in bathing should be guided by its effect on the system. If the cold bath in any form is speedily followed by a glow of warmth on the use of friction, such as a coarse towel, and increased strength, vigor and elasticity of spirits, it may be safely used. If, on the contrary, reaction is slow in taking place, and the bathing is followed by lassitude, debility, painful nervous excitement, or headache, it should be avoided.

Time of Bathing.—Early in the morning, or three or four hours after breakfast, are undoubtedly the best times for bathing. Cold bathing should, in no case, be indulged in immediately after a meal, for then it is necessary that the circulation should not be disturbed, as the stomach requires all its strength to digest the food. Three or four hours after breakfast the food is so far digested that the process will not be disturbed. Neither should the cold bath be indulged in when much fatigued, or after violent exercise, for at this time the power of reaction is reduced, and bad effects might be the result. If the power of evolving heat be entire, active, and continuous, no danger need be apprehended. But if a person is exhausted and weakened by exercise, if he is perspiring and rapidly parting with heat, if the exercise is over and he remains at rest during and immediately after the application of cold, then there is danger. The danger is not from the application of cold when the body is hot, but when the body is cooling, after having been heated.

In all those cases where death is occasioned by drinking cold water, it will be found that the body, heated and fatigued by exertion, was rapidly losing heat by profuse perspiration, the person having generally at the time closed his exertions. If the exertion had been continued, or at any rate the heat kept at its previous standard, no danger would have resulted. It was in this way that Alexander lost more of his army, than had ever been slain in his most bloody battle, when they, thirsty, weary and perspiring with their long march across the desert, rushed wildly into the cold waters of the river Oxus.

CLOTHING.

Clothing is an equivalent for a certain amount of food. There are some tribes, even in cold regions, who go almost naked, but they take a great deal of athletic exercise, and consume an enormous amount of carbon, in the form of meat and train-oil. The animal heat thus generated enables them to withstand the severity of the climate. In warm regions comfort requires the inhabitants to wear as little clothing, and that of as light a texture and fitting as loosely as possible.

It is usually advisable in our changeable northern climate

to wear flannel next the skin the year through. It protects the system from the rapid changes of temperature, the alternations of heat and cold, of wet and dry, so common in northern latitudes. Of course that for summer wear should be as thin as possible. In persons predisposed to rheumatic complaints, silk may be substituted for flannel with decided benefit. The electric qualities of the silk in these cases produces a healthy and invigorating action to the skin.

The best clothing to protect us from external heat or cold, is one that is a bad conductor of heat. A piece of iron and a woolen garment may be at the same temperature, yet the iron feels much colder, because it conducts the heat more rapidly from us, whilst woolen conducts the heat so slowly that less is abstracted. Cloth, the tissue of which is loose and porous, containing air in its interstices, is a worse conductor than closer stuffs. This is owing to air being a bad conductor, and hence we understand why furs and long napped woolens are the warmest.

The facility with which cloth imbibes, or gives off moisture, affects naturally their warmth. Linen imbibes moisture with great rapidity, and parts with it readily. It is therefore cooler than cotton or woolen, which imbibes moisture more slowly, gives it off more tardily, and can contain a considerable quantity without its being perceptible.

Bearing these facts in mind, we can more satisfactorily adapt our clothing to different climates, seasons, ages, and sexes.

The amount of clothing necessary for comfort, of course, every one must decide for himself. The power of resisting cold, or enduring heat, depends, as I have already stated, in a great degree upon the proper kind and amount of food, an active circulation and healthy digestion, lungs, and skin. When the circulation and the secretions of the system are active and healthy, the power of resisting cold is immense.

Every young man should have a certain amount of active exercise. If his food has been of the proper character, and his skin is in a healthy state, he is able to endure cold with much less clothing than those, who, pampered with luxuries, and constantly breathing heated air, too often, alas! poisoned with tobacco smoke, and reeking with the fumes of liquor, find it necessary to wear an immense amount of clothing to protect them from the cold. A sufficient amount of clothing should be worn to insure comfort, taking care to change it as the temperature requires, if it is twice a day. The chest covered by that portion of the linen which is exposed to view, should be protected by an additional thickness of flannel. For this portion of the chest is much more exposed than any other. In the covering of the throat, great care should be taken not to have it high, or fit too close. In either case the circulation to and from the head is impeded, and a man is liable to feel very decidedly the first sensations of hanging. Weakness and disease of the throat is not unfrequently induced by this practice. The best protection of the throat is to allow the hair upon the chin and throat to grow to at least two or three inches in length. The warmth and electric state of the hair protects the throat from changes of temperature, gives it additional strength, and prevents, in a great measure, those difficulties about the throat or voice which are so common in cold and damp weather. Clergymen, and those accustomed to much speaking and exposure, should not neglect these simple rules. Custom, when founded on reason, should be observed, but when it directs any class of men to divest themselves of the natural covering of the lower portion of the face and throat, the sooner it is disregarded the better.

Those garments next the skin should be frequently changed, otherwise the perspiration which is constantly passing from the system, saturates the garment and closes up the pores. Clothing worn during the day should not be worn at night. Stockings should be changed every day if possible. Very much depends on keeping the feet clean, dry, and healthy, as there is a singular sympathy between the cutaneous functions of the feet and other parts of the body. The feet should be warm, and the circulation active, or some other portion of the body, particularly the lungs, will be likely to suffer. Thick, double-soled boots, with double uppers, if well made, are much better protection to the feet than India-rubbers, which are apt to make the feet cold and damp.

Not only should damp stockings be speedily changed, but also damp or wet clothing, unless the person is keeping up active and vigorous exercise, when there is but little danger, as the amount of animal heat is not reduced. It is when the body is at rest, and therefore parting with heat, that the rapid abstraction of it by means of damp clothing, is prejudicial to health.

Additional garments, especially during the spring and fall, should be worn on going out in the evening, as the air is then usually more damp and chilly than during the day. Travelers accustomed to sleep at night, when journeying either by rail-car or stage, should always be provided with an extra cloak to wrap around them. It is during sleep, when the body is in a perfect state of repose, and its power of resisting external influences the smallest, that we are the most likely to take cold.

Color of clothing.—The color of our clothes is a subject well worthy of attention. White colors reflect the rays of heat, which are absorbed by the black. It is obvious that the color which renders the transmission of heat from without difficult, must equally impede the transmission of the heat of the body to without; and from these properties of colors, it will be manifest that white is better adapted for both summer and winter clothing.

As a general principle, then, clothes of light color may be regarded as adapted for every season and every climate.

There is another point connected with the color of the clothes, which, to persons whose duties often lead them into the sick room, or into miasmatic districts, is of vast importance. When pieces of cloth of different colors are exposed to the particles emanating from bodies, the dark colors absorb twice as much as the light. In times of contagious disease, then, black is the worst color that can be worn. Physicians formerly dressed in black, but after a time they began to understand that they had chosen the color of all others the most dangerous to themselves and patients. Contagious disease is often carried from one family to another in the clothes. Those whose duties lead them in the midst of infectious disease, should wear light clothing, as experience has shown that this color absorbs less of the emanations from the diseased body than others.

EXERCISE.

Judicious exercise contributes materially to physical development and sound health. The man accustomed to that kind of labor which brings into active exercise the muscles of the body, is usually well developed, the muscles hard, full and strong, and capable of long continued exertion. On the contrary, with those accustomed to but little physical labor, the muscles are usually more soft, the circulation less active, and the person more liable to fatigue.

The muscles consist of bundles of small fibers gradually changing towards the end into tendons or cords, by which they are strongly attached to the bones. The stimuli of the nerves acting on these fibers, causes them to contract and produce the varied and rapid movements of which the body is capable. The frequent contraction of these muscular fibers increases the flow of arterial blood towards them, and therefore develops them in size and strength. Every movement the system is capable of, is the result of the contraction of some muscle or set of muscles. The daring and almost miraculous feats of the equestrian, show the power and elasticity of the muscular system when fully trained and developed. Of course, where there is perfect health, all the organs of the body must be active; if tasked beyond their strength, or if but little is given them to do, weakness and disease will be the necessary consequence. If any organ is exerted too powerfully, too much arterial blood will be directed towards it, producing serious disturbance. Moderate exercise has a beneficial or tonic influence, whilst if it exceeds the bounds of moderation it may have an opposite result.

For the system to receive the full benefit of which it is capable from exercise, it should be combined with mental amusement. Much may depend upon the mere exercise of the muscles, and much upon the change of air, which attends many varieties of exercise ; but a combination of mental occupation and amusement with these is of high importance.

This is illustrated in the miserable experience of men who were once engaged in the habits of industrious trade, and whose success and wealth have encouraged and enabled them to retire from business. The monotony of every-day life is insupportable to them, and they resort to various forms of exercise for relief. The dumb-bell is tugged, and the feet and legs are dragged along the walks and avenues of a garden, but alike uselessly. They fail, because they want the pleasurable zest.

Walking is one of the gentlest forms of active exercise, when on a plain, and in moderation. The muscles of the body are exerted, but without exciting in them feelings of fatigue.

Dancing is a union of stepping and leaping. When used in moderation it constitutes an excellent exercise, besides communicating a grace and freedom to the motions, which they might not otherwise acquire. To those whose occupations are of a sedentary character, it is peculiarly appropriate.

Fencing is another excellent exercise. It brings into play particularly the muscles of the arms and chest, and indirectly every part of the body. Not only this, but it keeps the mind actively employed, for it requires a considerable amount of skill to parry the rapid thrusts of an adroit fencer. Riding on horseback, swimming, and skating, are among the most fascinating and healthful exercises with which we are acquainted. The skater gliding over the smooth surface of the ice, presents in his swift movements a perfect picture of manly grace and beauty. A knowledge of swimming, independent of the benefit derived from exercise in the water, is often the means of saving life.

These athletic sports and manly exercises, should form a part of every young man's education. Gymnastic exercises should not be forgotten by those of sedentary pursuits. There are innumerable aches and pains, which would rapidly vanish, if the circulation were quickened by a little judicious use of the muscles. I refer now, of course, to those whose every day duties require but little out-door exercise.

The proper development of the chest contributes, not only to manly beauty, but wards off those terrific diseases, which, fastening their talons in the lungs and heart, poison the fountains of life and drag the victim down slowly, it may be, but surely to death. Exercise of the muscles of the chest, keeping the shoulders thrown back, and drawing in the breath slowly, so that all the air cells of the lungs may be filled, increases materially the strength and size of the chest and lungs. If we add to this a proper cultivation and judicious use of the voice, both in speaking and singing, filling the chest with air, and letting the tones of the voice flow out full, clear and distinct, we have a powerful preventive to the development of disease of the chest.

As we have before said, a person should not sit down immediately after violent exercise, to a hearty meal, but should give the weakened system a few moments to rally ; neither should he commence active labor as soon as he has swallowed his food, but allow the stomach a few moments to direct its entire powers to the digestion of its contents.

CHAPTER III.

CULTIVATION OF MORAL AND INTELLECTUAL FACULTIES.

We have glanced, in the preceding chapter, at the physiological structure of man, and the healthy development of his physical powers. Let us now look at the moral and intellectual powers.

We know that we all have have within us germs of good, faculties which, if rightly cultivated, make us in harmony with the purity and truth of the God of nature and love. The proper training and cultivation of these faculties develop all that is manly, pure, and noble within us, expand the soul, and shed around us the genial warmth and influence which ever flows from the good. Were there no hereafter, and were that fearful maxim true, once written over the gateway of a city of the dead, "Death is an eternal sleep," still would the happiness of man be found in the paths of purity and truth.

In all ages of the world, from the time that sin first stained the earth to the present, has the violation of moral or physical laws brought their own fearful penalty, even here in this life. We cannot violate the laws of our being with impunity, even if we would, for the evil results flowing from their disobedience, follow as naturally as day follows night.

To be healthy, to be great and noble, and be remembered with love and veneration by the good, our being must be like an instrument, in which there shall be no discordant note or jarring string, but all the faculties of the mind so happily blended, so harmonious in action, as to form one perfect whole. The more nearly we approximate to this standard, the more shall we have fulfilled the great end of our being.

Our passions were given us for use, but reason was also given us to keep them under proper control. A cold, passionless man, would be the most forlorn and unlovable object in the world. Pride, strongly developed, and the ruling dominant principle of life, renders one like ice surrounded by its own freezing atmosphere, an atmosphere which would chill a warm and genial soul. And thus, from the undue development of any one passion or faculty of the mind, the most fearful evils and desolating vices have been introduced into the human family. War, steeping the earth in blood, and crushing the living beneath its grinding taxations,—vice, hydra-headed, poisoning the fountains of life, rearing the gibbet, building high, and broad, and strong the prison wall, and that dark and fearful catalogue of crimes which have changed men into demons, and made the heavens echo with the wail of suffering and agony, going up in all ages of the world from thousands of crushed and bleeding hearts—are all developed from this lack of harmony in ourselves, in this cultivation, or giving free scope to one set of passions or feelings to the exclusion of all others.

True greatness can only be achieved by developing the whole being. The first step in this great plan of physical and intellectual development is, of course, in the nursery—and the first teacher, the mother. Well will it be for the child in after life if that mother understands her responsibility, and seeks to develop the good and noble in its nature, and check, with gentle hand, the first half-unconscious step in the path of wrong. The child will need, as he ascends the scale of life and mingles, in his boyhood, with the world, all a mother's pure and holy teachings, all that love of virtue, purity, and truth, which the loving mother instils into the mind of her child, to shield it from the vices of the world. And those vices meet him at every step, lure him with winning smiles and honeyed words into their embrace, weave around him the meshes of their silken net, and scattering his pathway with flowers, and entrancing his senses with the witching smiles of beauty and the harmony of music, bind him hand and foot in chains stronger than iron, tainting the purity of his soul, and the fountains of life, with the leprosy of death. When the boy reaches the age of puberty, and feels stirring within the strength and passions of manhood, he finds no lack of teachers to give him his initiatory lessons of vice,—vices which, oh! how often! change the bright sparkle of the eye and the joyous laugh, to the dull, leaden stare, and the painful laugh of idiocy or insanity.

Vices to which the Young are Exposed.—First and foremost among the young in almost every grade of society, among the high and the low, the rich and the poor, the educated and refined, and particularly in our schools and colleges, we notice the development of that fearful vice, *self pollution.* First practiced, before the fearful consequences are understood, it is oftentimes persisted in until the poor victim is reduced to idiocy or insanity, or driven into an early grave. Its effects upon the system are pernicious in the extreme, prostrating the vital powers, and affecting, in a powerful degree, the brain, the nervous system, the organs of digestion and secretion. This will readily be perceived, when it is understood that the arterial blood flows through its appropriate artery into the organs of generation, and furnishes the materials for the formation of *semen.* The semen is formed from the very life of the blood, and its constant formation draws from the system more powerfully its vital force, than would be the case if an artery was opened and as much blood as was required to form the semen was permitted to flow out; for, in the former case, in addition to the abstraction of the vital fluid, is the powerful action produced in the formation of the semen, upon the brain and nervous system.

This practice long persisted in is sure to leave its sad marks upon the mind as well as the body. The eye assumes a lack-lustre expression; the face sometimes becomes pale and covered with pimples; there is a lassitude, or a fretfulness and peevishness of disposition, or a total disregard of the affections of life. The digestion is impaired, the circulation sluggish, and the face rapidly assumes the wrinkled expression of age. Soon there is perceptible a blunting of the finer feelings of the nature, society is avoided for the luxury of secret practice, the senses become obtuse, the sparkle of the mind is gone, a slow decline of all the mental faculties, ending in death, or the living death of idiocy or insanity closes the scenes.

This habit is even indulged among children, who are initiated not unfrequently, by servants or their young companions. In all cases, however, whether the practice is commenced either before or after puberty, if persisted in, it develops a long train of difficulties, such as weakness of the genital organs, impotence, and all that torturing train of diseases which accompany impaired digestion and deranged vital power, and sows in the system the seeds of death.

Upon how many households this blighting curse falls, dragging down the child of beauty and of promise, and, unmindful of the agonizing tears of parents, instils the poison of death where, before, all was purity and fragrance, the records of the grave alone can show.

Strange as it may seem, the free indulgence in this vice generally develops a positive dislike for female society, so that its victims are seldom found among the haunts of prostitution. But the wide portals of these palaces of sin are thronged by hosts of others, who, in the sparkling wine cup and the excitement of sensual passions, are forgetting their manhood, and staining their souls with sin.

Gambling and licentiousness.—Thronging the dark pathway of evil, and bound together by unseen influences, are the *drinking saloon, gambling hells,* and the *halls of revelry and licentious debauch.* Vice is garlanded with flowers. It lies concealed amid the gorgeous beauties of art, the blandishments and smiles of beauty, and the intoxicating charms of music. How brightly foams and sparkles the wine-cup, how softly gleam the lights, and how brightly the mirrors reflect from their dazzling surfaces forms of physical beauty and grace! Step by step along that charmed pathway the victim glides. The finer, holier feelings of his nature are blunted. The mad excitement of gambling absorbing every faculty of the mind, opens wide the door to a vast throng of feelings and practices, which at length may close around him the cold walls of a prison, and send him an outcast from society. Late suppers and the free indulgence of the wine-cup among young men is like to throw them into society not the most select or pure in their feelings and practices. This class of dissipation impairs the digestion, robs the system of its vital force, and shortens the length of human life. It also often makes easy the path to licentious excesses.

Remember that in New York alone there are nearly twenty thousand who eat their bread from the wages of prostitution. What a vast throng to prey upon society! Some clad in silks and satins, some clothed in rags; some in the first flush of womanhood, with the blush of shame yet tinging their cheeks, some in the rounded fullness of voluptuous beauty, with winning smiles and honeyed words, and others in rags and filth, with disease fearful and disgusting eating away their life. Some of the fruits of this vice are immediate, filling the body with suffering, and oftentimes making a person an object of loathing, even to himself. Walk for one short hour the wards of a hospital, and see the loathsome ravages of disease in varied forms produced by this vice. The eye sickens at the painful sight, and you turn away in wonder that man can so far forget his self-respect, as to sink so low. But these are only a specimen of cases where the effects of disease are apparent to the sight. But who shall lift the curtain and show the vast throng with tainted souls and poisoned blood, transmitting as a sad heritage the fruits of their follies to future generations.

Rest assured that violations of moral law will not go unpunished, even in this world. What though you may escape the taint of physical disease, and the sad fate of cursing coming generations with its poison, what can restore the purity and freshness of the mind, what compensate for loss of self-respect? Licentious indulgence blunts the finer feelings of the heart, and if persisted in, even without the aid of those vices which accompany it like loving friends, turns the heart into a charnel-house of pure affections. But the awful fruit of this and kindred vices are confined not to the present, but extend through life and develop themselves in a bitter harvest in generations yet unborn.

I have spoken of these vices becaused they have rolled their chilling waves over many a child of promise, blasted the fairest hopes, bowed down the grey head of age, and wrung tears of blood from many a wife and mother. Oh, drunkenness, licentiousness and gambling, could death yield from its cold grasp that mighty throng whom you have sent to the welcome embrace of the grave ; could the cells of the insane, and prison walls restore your victims to the world, oh ! what sad faces, what crowds of broken-hearts would meet our gaze !

I have spoken of these vices, because they beset the paths of men, open wide their doors, and invite the unwary to enter; and because I know, for I have seen the awful wrecks they have made, that when once within their grasp, their influence is often overwhelming.

Healthful Development of the Mind.—There are always, for the well-cultivated mind, ample, healthful amusements, easily obtained, and which leave no sting behind. In the resources of a well-cultivated mind there are stores of enjoyment which can never enter the conception of the ignorant. Nature is all alive and radiant with beauty. Every twinkling star studding the diadem of night, every tree, every flower, and every drop of water, speaks in familiar language. The great storehouse of nature is opened, and the delighted mind wanders at will among its glories and its beauties. History unlocks the records of tho past, and the great and good who have lived in all ages re-appear on the stage, and move in grand and solemn beauty before us. Who would wish to steep his soul in vice, when nature, everywhere, in all its works, teaches purity and truth, and when his path is strewed with wrecks and ruins of men, and the voice of nations comes up mournfully and sad through the night of ages, telling the vices which led to their downfall?

The more the mind is trained to active and vigorous thought, the more will it be enabled to grapple with the great problems of life, and make its influence felt on the world around. In this age of action, when mind is everywhere pluming its wings for daring flights, the clear and vigorous intellects leave their mark upon the age, or, in the more quiet walks of life, are respected and beloved by those who are striving with them to fulfill life's great mission.

Far more rational enjoyment is furnished in the reading-room, the library, and the lecture-room, than in any of the paths of dissipation. The mind is amused, strengthened, and furnished food for thought, and the healthy action of the system undisturbed. This cannot be said of those who, night after night, breathe the heated and poisonous air of drinking saloons, whose passions are inflamed by drink, gambling, or sensual indulgence, and who gradually learn to delight in vulgar jokes and conversation. The nervous system is deranged, the organs of digestion impaired, and the harmony of the system destroyed. The bitter fruit, in some form or other, will sooner or later be gathered. Abused or violated nature will speak, in suffering, in derangement of the functions of life, and in shortening the path to the grave.

The charms of social life should not be disregarded. The plodding student, or man of business, who never unbends from his stern duties, and who thinks all pleasant social conversation a waste of time, looses the zest, the sparkle and poetry of life. The social circle and the pleasant converse of friends, are the green spots along the dusty path of life, where the mind, refreshed and invigorated, is made strong for action, and contented with its daily duties. There is a peculiar charm in refined and intelligent ladies' society. There is in them a polish, a refinement and delicacy of mind, a spiritual beauty and grace, which, brought in contact with the sterner sex, does much to humanize and refine them. Fortunate is that man who has had a mother's kind teachings, and the sweet society of sisters.

All those who have a fondness for beauty, purity, and truth, who love to linger amid the warm sunshine and sweet flowers of life, find increasing stores of delight in the beauties of art, in the bright gems of literature, and in the wonders of nature. The glories of art seem to uplift them into a higher and purer atmosphere—into a world of the ideal and spiritual. Literature brings them in contact with the burning, flashing minds of genius in all ages of the world; elevating the soul, developing and ripening the better feelings of our nature. The honey bee, from the flowers of the most poisonous plants, extracts the sweetest honey. The human mind, in which the principle of purity and truth is strongly developed, who looks upon the human family as one great brotherhood, ever moving on toward that spirit-world, where the wronged will be righted, where earth's disguises will be swept away, and the naked workings of the spirit stand revealed to every eye, can see in the midst of the wrong, the misery, and degradation around him, flowers trampled to the earth, which only require the helping hand of human sympathy and kindness to enable them to lift up their heads and again shed their fragrance on the air.

Plant not your heel upon the prostrate; taunt not the fallen with their folly; wrap not yourself around with the mantle of your own righteousness; nor pass by on the other side, while the lips curl in scorn, and you say, "touch me not, for I am holier than thou." You know not the fearful storm through which they may have passed—how their hopes in life may have been blasted—how temptation may have beset their path—how they have sunk lower and lower, until they have become objects of loathing and scorn—festering sores upon the bosom of society.

Try, by your example and your practice, to stay that mighty tide of evil which is desolating society, rolling its lava flood over the brightest, fairest flowers in earth's garden

—piling the earth with graves, and making the heavens above us echo with the sighs and the groans of the heart-broken, the wronged, and the suffering. Shun, as you would the breath of the pestilence, those destroyers of men—those contemners of virtue—those fiends disguised as men, who, with hearts callous to pity, would lead you along with honeyed words and flowery chains, until you find the chains have become fetters of iron, and the holy, the pure, and the true, the noble and God-like within you are withering away in that burning, poisonous breath around you.

Remember, in the gay revel, when the wine-cup foams and sparkles—when the mad excitement of gambling is fastening upon you—when beauty smiles and invites you to illicit pleasures—when, amid the excitement of business, you seek to defraud your neighbor, or oppress the poor, the widow, and the orphan—that there is danger in playing with the asp; that, for a violation of moral laws, a day of reckoning will assuredly come—even in this life. If not in sickness and disease, it will in the choking up of the gushing springs of love and tenderness, in a barrenness of the heart's affections.

The mind, taught to look on life as it is, can glean lessons of instruction from almost every page. His reason and his judgment will tell him that the drama is not all corrupt, and that golden lessons may be taught from the stage. The novel, properly selected, he may read in his leisure hours, with profit, for, in the form of a tale, in proper hands, the most searching analysis of motives may be given, and mighty truths and holy thoughts scattered broadcast over the world. His discriminating mind may select the good, and cast the bad away. There will be no affinity in his mind towards books, dramas, or men, obscene or demoralizing in their teachings.

I have endeavored, in this chapter, to show that happiness, health, and true greatness, are only obtained in obedience to moral and physical laws. The higher are our aspirations for the true and the beautiful, the more will our minds become developed, the clearer, more powerful and active will be our intellect—the more shall we be in harmony with nature—and the greater our influence for good upon the world. And more than this, violations of these laws of our being bring with them, in this world, their own fearful penalty, in sickness, disease, and death—in a deadening of the sensibilities—in a deterioration or stagnation of intellect—or a mind like a ruined instrument, with here and there a brilliant note intermingled with hideous discords.

We now proceed to speak of matrimony, viewed in the light of reason, as an institution we should view not alone through the medium of passion and the gorgeous romance of love, but in the calm, clear light of reason and of truth, looking forward into the future as well as the present.

MARRIAGE.

Marriage, as originally designed by our Creator, is a law of our being. There is no period of our life when we are independent of others for our happiness. The child is shielded from want by the strong arms of its parents. As we step from childhood on to the stage of action, the wife clings confidingly to her husband, and the husband turns for sympathy to the warm heart of the wife, and gathers courage and strength, to meet the duties of life, from her cheering smiles. As we descend into second childhood, when time gradually whitens our heads, dims our eyes, and renders our steps uncertain, then we love to lean on those over whose childhood we watched, and our children lighten our pathway to the grave.

Marriage, however, in these degenerate days, when iniquity and corruption are abroad in the world, and the fountains of life, in many an instance, are tainted with disease, should not be consummated in haste or in a reckless spirit, but only after mature deliberation. That romance of love, which endows the object of adoration with the charms and virtues of angels and of gods, which can see no faults, and can dream of nothing but Eden bliss, may, by-and-by, become chilled. When reality begins to take the place of romance, possibly a frown may appear upon that angel face, and from those ruby lips flow tones *not* of the sweetest music; and, as the illusion gradually disappears, there may be found an entire absence of those essential qualifications for happiness, without which the home becomes cold and cheerless. A family, where all is discord and contention, gives about as good a foretaste of hell as one can well have.

The relation between husband and wife is one of the

most sacred, and should be the most perfect and harmonious, of any in life. The man who enters into it carelessly, or blinded and intoxicated by passion, may regret his folly through life. Other things should be taken into consideration, aside from the blind impulses of passion, or the cool calculations of wealth or position in society.

Every sensible man, who marries, hopes to have children, and to be surrounded with some of the comforts and charms of a home. There are those who marry a fortune, and look upon the wife as a necessary incumbrance, but they can hardly be ranked among sensible men.

That the home may be made happy, and the children grow up in health and vigor of intellect, not only must harmony reign within the domestic circle, but certain laws of our nature must be obeyed.

Time of Marriage.—No positive rule can be laid down as to proper time for marriage. In warm climates, people are much more rapidly developed than in colder regions. In equatorial countries, menstruation may take place as early as ten years of age, and it is not uncommon to see fathers and mothers not more than twelve or thirteen years of age. As we go into colder regions the young reach puberty at a much later period, varying from fourteen to twenty years of age.

In our temperate climates, we may safely say that the male should not contract marriage before the age of twenty-five, nor the females before twenty. There are, of course, exceptions to this rule; but, as a general thing, it will be found that early marriages are followed by unhealthy children, if not in infancy, still lacking that strength and vigor of constitution which will enable them to live to a healthy old age. Aside from this, when the wife steps almost from the nursery into the arms of her husband, she lacks maturity of form and that physical strength which will enable her to tread calmly, and with self-reliance, the thorny path of life. Marriage, in these cases, is apt to be followed by a long train of sufferings, by a broken down constitution, and an early death. In both sexes the system should be fully matured before marriage. Excessive exertion of any part of the body before complete development has taken place, is succeeded by fatigue or decay of such part. Hence it is obvious that marriage, at too early an age, or the premature exertion of the genital functions, must not only be highly injurious to the parents, in most cases, but also to the constitution of the offspring. To accomplish the great end of marriage—the propagation of healthful infants—both male and female should observe the strictest continence until the adult age.

The ancient Germans did not marry until the twenty-fourth or twenty-fifth year, previous to which they observed the most rigid chastity ; in consequence of which their offspring acquired a size and strength that excited the astonishment of Europe. Precocious sexual intercourse greatly debilitates the moral, intellectual, and physical powers of both sexes, producing diminished growth and strength of the male, delicate and bad health of the female, premature old age or death of either or both, and a feeble and scrofulous offspring.

Louis XI. cohabited before the age of fourteen with his queen, who was not twelve ; and his effeminate and ferocious character undoubtedly depended, in some degree, on the exhaustion of his nascent powers. Our daily intercourse with the world, shows that neither in the male nor female does the mind or body acquire perfectibility until many years after puberty. The young man, with the down of childhood still on his cheeks, could communicate but very little vigor or vitality to his offspring. The constitution, also, of the young mother, would be very likely to be broken down by the disorders of pregnancy, and the fatigue of labor and suckling. More than this, at this early age, the moral and physical states are not fully developed ; and the impetuous exercise of ungovernable passion, and the facilities for prolonging it, would lead to satiety, disgust, and debility.

We not unfrequently see boys and girls at the head of families, just about as fit to perform the duties devolving upon them, as when they were in their nurse's arms. Their happiness for life, the health of the mother as well as the prosperity of the father, may be wrecked by their early marriage and the consequences. Rest assured, the duties and cares of life will come soon enough, and will require, to meet them as they should be met, more than the strength, the skill, and judgment, which usually fall to the lot of childhood.

The consequences of premature marriages are more to

be dreaded when men have previously led dissipated lives, passing, as it were, through a period of fifty years in sixteen.

If too early a marriage has a tendency to produce unhealthy children, so, also, has a marriage contracted late in life, when the re-productive power is deficient in vigor. Unfortunately, men frequently live until they are forty-five or fifty before marriage, and are then connected with those much younger than themselves. The consequence, as a general thing, is, feeble children, who often die prematurely.

Suitableness of Age.—A considerable disproportion between the ages of parents, is another fruitful cause, not only of unhealthful offspring, but of ill health on the part of one or both the parents. In a judicious marriage, there should be but a few years difference between the ages of the parties. Old age cannot wed with youth, with the expectation of harmony in the domestic circle, or of vigorous and healthy offspring, any more than winter can mingle with summer. Flowers look sickly, and are chilled by winter, and so is youth when united to age. The young should not sleep with the aged, though the difference may not be more than fifteen or twenty years, for the vital power in the young is rapidly exhausted by the aged. For the same reason, the cold and phlegmatic temperament should not sleep with one of warm and nervous temperament, for a similar result is produced. The manifest difference in age, temperament, and constitution, where the parties are placed in so close a relation, are pregnant with disastrous results to the weak and young, as well, if the parties are married, to their offspring.

In marriage, as a general thing, the husband should be the oldest, although the difference should never amount to more than ten or fifteen years, and four or five would be still better. If a girl unites herself in marriage with a man old enough to be her father, we feel that there is a violation of nature's laws; but, when we see a young man leading to the altar a lady old enough to be his mother, we can hardly refrain from feeling pity for both.

Harmony of Feeling to be Considered in Marriage.—Marriage is not a light act, to gratify and while away an idle hour, but an institution whose influences extend through unborn generations. If rightly consummated, in obedience to the design of the Creator, it is the most happy relation which can exist in the world.

The great question for a young man to decide, in selecting a partner for life, is not worldly wealth, for a man can have but little spirit, and but poorly understand his mission, if he is willing to settle down in idleness on his wife's fortune; neither should he be anxious to trace her ancestral lineage back to barbarian times, or seek to find her among the gay frivolities of fashionable life, for he may afterwards find, to his sorrow, that fashionable life is, sometimes, but another name for dissipation and heartlessness.

He should rather seek to know whether she has those sterling qualities of mind and heart which will shed a bright and genial warmth over his home, and gladden his heart by her cheerful soul, her purity and truth. Many a man has found the better feelings of his nature crippled, and the generous, the noble, and lofty aspirations of his soul, chilled by a selfish, bigoted, or ignorant wife. With the ability to soar upward, like the lark, into the pure air and bright sunlight of Heaven, he is kept by her influence so near the earth, that, like the swallow, the wings of his spirit are bedrabbled with its mire and filth.

A pretty face, a graceful form, and sparkling wit, may so entrance the senses as to exclude everything like reason, and make the man rush blindly and headlong, without further thought, into the arms of matrimony. After marriage, reality is likely to take the place of romance, and the poor fellow may find that, in fluttering about the candle, he has singed his wings in the flame.

There should be, in married life, a harmony of feeling, a blending together of soul, a perfect confidence in the purity and integrity of the other. With this, the marriage state is a bright foretaste of the union of souls in the spirit-world. With a faithful heart and sympathizing soul at home, a man can bear up against the trials of life, and bravely battle with its storms and tempests. But, destroy this confidence, let the home be cold and cheerless, with no gushing forth of the heart's more tender feelings, with discord and contention, fretfulness and repining, and the charm of home is gone. It ceases to be a quiet resting-place amid the troubled waters of life, and drags the soul earthward, by the development of evil passions, when it should have been borne upwards on the strong, yet gentle wings of love.

A proper harmony of feeling—the wife respecting the husband, and the husband the wife, the souls of both flowing and mingling together, forming a beautiful unit in thought, in affection, and interest—leaves its impress not only on their own characters, but on that of their children. Children are quick in their perceptions, and a frowning look or a harsh word between their parents, although apparently unnoticed, still leaves its mark for evil on the forming mind. As years roll on, and the mind of the child becomes more developed, so do those wrangling scenes in the home circle, or those cold and sneering words and the heartlessness and barrenness of affection which, alas! is so often found there, produce its fearful influence in the development of its character.

Let the home be the dearest, brightest, spot on earth, and the lessons there taught be those of purity and truth, of harmony and love. How often, alas! where parties are united with no affinity for each other, is it made a school for evil. Need we wonder, when we look abroad upon the earth, and see the crime which everywhere lifts its head, and the vices which taint the current of society, when we know that, in the majority of cases, the first lessons were taught in the sanctuary of home? That want of harmony, wrangling, and discord there, have developed those evil passions in the child, which, going on unchecked, have gained a mastery over the thoughts and feelings, and, at length, filled the prisons with victims, and society with heartlessness, vice, and crime.

Until the institution of marriage is rightly understood, in all its relations and all its duties, and the parties guided in their selection by reason, judgment, and honesty, and integrity of purpose, we may build our asylums in vain; in vain may the clergy hurl the anathemas of God against vice, it will still lift its head in our midst, still roll its cold and chilling tide over many a home, over many a bleeding, breaking heart.

But, if there are duties the wife owes to the husband, there are, also, duties the husband owes to the wife. Man, is the sturdy oak, drawing sustenance and strength from the mother earth, and from the light and air of Heaven; woman, the tender vine, clinging to him with her tendrils, and enfolding him in the green foliage of her pure and deathless love. Beware how you rend those tendrils—how you tear from you that green foliage and scatter it in the dust. It is a sad thing to see a woman wither and die as she, alas! too often, dies, of a broken heart! She may not have been faultless, yet stung by ingratitude, by neglect, by unfaithfulness, by cold and sneering words, she may have withered away and died; or, goaded to desperation, she may have become reckless of life, and rushed madly into dissipation or crime. Pause before you condemn her too strongly. Ask your own heart who has been the most fearfullly to blame?

Constitution and Temperament.—As we have before said, one of the great objects of marriage is to become parents. In selecting a wife, then, the constitution, temperament, general health, and hereditary predisposition to disease, should be taken into consideration. If the man is of a weak and scrofulous constitution, a union with one of the same constitution would be followed by disastrous results in the children. The unhealthy current of life flowing both from father and mother, and meeting in the child, would either materially shorten its life, or be very liable to make its existence one of suffering. For the same reason those nearly related to each other should not be united in marriage, for any elements of disease existing in one, would be almost sure to exist in the other—thus rendering the propagation of healthy children impossible. But, aside from this, the union of near relatives would of itself be sufficient to produce unhealthy children, oftentimes feeble in intellect. It is from this system of intermarriages that some of the royal families of Europe have become almost idiotic.

A union, without affection, or the old united with the young, will also cause the children to be scrofulous, and be likely to shorten their lives.

Mercenary considerations, in many instances, lead to marriage. How often is the decrepitude of age, or the unhealthy girl, who has grown up like a hot-house plant, without vigor, either of body or intellect, preferred to the strong and healthy, of modest and virtuous conduct, when unconnected with a weighty purse? Can we expect, in these cases, a happy domestic circle, or a healthy progeny? Those who thus violate nature's laws may repent, in long years of suffering, their fool-hardy temerity.

Generation of Organized Beings.—Every animal and plant has derived its vitality from its parents, and these from their ancestors, retrogading in succession, to the creation of organized matter by the Supreme Being. Reproduction consists in the growth of an ovum, germ, seed, or embryo, in a living part, from which it is separated when capable of independent existence. The females of plants and animals supply the germ—the males secrete a fluid, which, placed in contact with this, fecundates or vivifies it. Plants and animals must acquire a certain development before they can reproduce their species.

Organized beings have three periods of life—youth, the age of generation, and that of senescence or sterility. The period of generation is accelerated by warm climates and stimulating nutriment, and cut short by a variety of causes. A female does not conceive after the cessation of the menses, which usually occurs between the age of forty-five and fifty; and yet men of vigorous constitutions are, sometimes, capable of reproduction at the age of ninety, or even a hundred. Men often abuse the generative functions; they consume their vitality, exhaust themselves, and often, by their excessive indulgence, produce premature old age or death.

Long continued debauchery, whether with women or by masturbation, will cause impotence. Every exciting or depressing passion, which operates during the act of reproduction, may be a temporary cause of impotence. All causes of debility, whether moral or physical, impede the function of generation.

Long watching, great fatigue mental or corporeal, want of nutriment, excessive evacuations sanguinous or otherwise, malignant fever, diseases of the brain and spinal marrow whether from external injuries or poisons, and numerous other diseases, are temporary causes of impotence. The abuses of narcotics, such as tobacco and opium, of saline refrigerants, acids, iodine, camphor and nitre, are causes of impotence, as they reduce the muscular power below the ordinary state.

From what has been already said, it will readily be perceived that to conceive vigorous and healthy children, both in body and intellect, there must be not only healthy parents, but parents who, in their union, have not violated nature's laws. As the child derives its vitality from its parents, it will be either robust and active, as the parents were strong and healthy in their physical organization, or weak and feeble, as the parents lacked vitality, and as their blood had become tainted by disease and impurities, developed either by their own folly, or inherited from their ancestors. We cannot expect healthy children from weak and feeble parents, with a multitude of aches and pains, who transmit, with the life they impart to their offspring, the impurities and weakness of their own physical organizations.

Most men who become illustrious by character, genius, or valor, were the fruit of ardent and vigorous love, and the sons of parents who were either remarkable for physical strength, or for harmony of mind or refinement of feelings. Persons of strong and sound constitutions beget healthful infants—while those who make excessive mental or corporeal exertions have generally feeble offspring. It is for this reason that the simple rustic, robust and vigorous, may beget infants of high physical and moral powers; while men of the greatest genius, who over exert their mental faculties, often engender infants feeble both in mind and body.

Prolonged continence, in healthy parents, has a healthy effect on the child. The father of Montaigne returned after thirty-two years from the wars of Italy, was, during that period, strictly continent, and begat his celebrated son. The father of J. J. Rousseau returned from Constantinople, after a considerable absence, and brought to his spouse the reward of a long fidelity. Thus, by protracted continence, and purity of morals, the species are improved and strengthened, both in mind and body. Virtuous parents concentrate all the energy of their mind in abandoning themselves to the views of nature. They engender a posterity by whose talents the pride and glory of their progenitors will be maintained. Thus it is that, after many progressive and virtuous generations, we see families ennoble themselves and flourish ; but, by a subsequent incontinence, they fade and degenerate.

It is impossible to generate healthy children when the vigor and tono of the system is weakened by dissipation or constant sexual indulgence, or when the generative functions are excited by artificial stimuli. If the parents strive to obey the laws of their being, keeping their passions under proper restraint, their mind healthy, and their bodies vigorous and active, all the powers of nature are concentrated in the act, and a nervous force, a strength of vitality is imparted to the germ, which, in the womb of the mother, is to be developed into the living child.

Remember, that in the brief time allotted to us in this life, we must, if we fulfill the great end of our existence, develop the higher and nobler qualities of the soul, seek to uplift the race, bring it nearer God and more in harmony with His works, rather than plunge it still lower in the depths of moral and physical weakness and degradation. Not until men and women understand the true and sacred import of the marriage relation, looking upon it, not as a means for the acquisition of wealth, for display, or the gratification of sensual passions, but as a union of soul, an expanding of their higher faculties, a union in which, respecting the laws of their being, they shall bless, instead of curse, coming generations, will this tide of crime, which now desolates the earth, be stayed, and the corrupt current of life be purified. Then shall the human race, casting aside the fetters of its degradation and its sin-defiled garments, start into new life, and drawing nearer to God, be pervaded by the harmony of His spirit, and irradiated by the brightness and the glow of the spirit world.

CHAPTER IV.

INFLUENCE OF CLIMATE ON HEALTH.

THE beneficial effect of a change of climate in persons weak and debilitated, or suffering from some disease slow in its progress, and yet if allowed to go on unchecked, ending in death, is often strikingly apparent. The good results are not owing alone to a change of climate, but also to a change of scene, turning the mind into a different channel and developing new thoughts and feelings. The person who has always lived in a level country, or those whose lives have been spent amid the busy throng of a crowded city, find ever-varying and never-tiring scenes of pleasure in the ocean, in its calm stillness and in its angry power; in the grand and majestic scenery of a mountainous district, presenting as it does a combination of the grand and the beautiful, permitting the eye to take in at a single glance the rich luxuriance of spring, and the cold, dazzling whiteness of winter snows. The mind is refreshed and invigorated, the current of the blood is warmed and quickened, the eyes sparkle with a new life, and tho cheeks glow with a healthier hue.

There is a time, however, in the progress of disease, when home is the best place, and when it is cruelty on the part of physician or friends to draw the patient away from its quiet and its comforts, to be subject to the annoyance of travel, to mingle in new scenes and meet with strange faces. It is sad to die far away from one's native land, with no loving hand to smooth the dying pillow and wipe away those cold drops with which the brow is besprinkled from the river of death, as the soul passes over its icy waters to the spirit land.

When the system is very much weakened by disease, lengthy journeys should only be taken after mature deliberation and reliable medical advice. When, however, the system is prostrated by long-continued mental or physical labor, or disease is commencing its undermining influence, relaxation from business, and a change of climate and scene, will not unfrequently be of far more benefit than all the medicines the most skillful physician could suggest. The beneficial effects are very marked in that class of persons whose ancestors for several generations have lived in the same locality. In these cases, if the patient is residing in an inland place, a change to the seashore, or if living by the seashore, a few months spent in an inland place, where, notwithstanding it might be in the same latitude, there would still be an entire change of air, will often be followed by very decided benefit.

In that large class of persons who are merely suffering from a residence in the city, and close application to business, without any decided disease, the mere change to the country, either permanently or for a summer residence, may be all that is necessary to restore health. But to the invalid whose sufferings are occasioned by some particular *disease*, the selection of his temporary residence is of great moment. For one, an elevated situation, and a dry, bracing air, will be most proper; another will require a sheltered residence with a milder air; while the sea-side may be the situation indicated for the third.

The idea is prevalent, to a certain extent, that the beneficial effects of climate are evinced chiefly in consumptive diseases. This opinion is decidedly erroneous. In dyspepsia, and disorders of the digestive organs generally, and in the nervous disorders which so often accompany them; in asthma, in bronchial diseases, in scrofula, and in rheumatism, the beneficial effects of climate are even more marked than in consumption. In cases, also, of general delicacy of constitution and derangement of the system in childhood and in youth, which cannot be strictly classed under any of these diseases, and in that disordered state of the general health which so often occurs at a certain period of more advanced life, *climacteric disease*, in which the powers of the constitution, both mental and bodily, fail, and the system lapses into a state of premature decay, change of climate becomes a valuable remedial agent.

Change of Climate in Pulmonary Consumption.—Unfortunately for the patient, the incipient steps of this insidious disease are often overlooked, and not until violent cough, difficult breathing, and spitting of blood appear, is the patient or his friends alarmed. At this time he may have passed that point in his disease where he would be benefited by travel, leaving him but little to expect from a long journey but increased suffering and an early fatal termination. It is in the incipient stages of this fearful malady, before its fangs become deeply fastened in the system, that benefit is to be expected from change of air or scene. But when the disease has made rapid progress, and there are unmistakable evidences of extensive tuberculous deposit, the patient had better remain amid the comforts of home and the watchful care of friends. There are, however, cases of chronic consumption where the tuberculous affection is limited to a small portion of the lungs. These cases may, undoubtedly, be much relieved, if not entirely cured, by residing for a time in a mild climate, when aided by proper medicines and regimen.

There is no spot in this world, however soft the air, or bright the skies, where the climate can be said to be perfect; for a climate to be perfect in relation to consumption, should not vary in temperature from day to day throughout the year; and the transition from day to night, as well as from one season to the other, should be imperceptible. As such a climate does not exist, it only remains for us to find one which approaches nearest *equality* of temperature, for in that quality consists the chief virtue of climates as regards pulmonary complaints. The degree of heat is a very inferior consideration as compared with the range of temperature, and there is no reason why the mild, humid, relaxing atmosphere of Rome, or some of the West India

Islands, should be more efficacious, in the treatment of consumption, than the cold, rarefied air of Siberia, if the temperature of the latter were equable. A sea voyage in the early stage of the disease is often of very decided benefit. Persons troubled with cough, and other symptoms, which point unmistakably to the development of serious troubles, often find on the ocean, as they go into a different climate, all their old symptoms leaving them, and not unfrequently reach the end of their voyage perfectly restored to health.

If, then, a sea-voyage is decided upon, and a sojourn for a time in some foreign climate, the question arises, which among the various places of resort is the most desirable for a winter's residence.

The climate in the South of France is not a desirable residence for a consumptive invalid. Nice, is subject to great alterations from heat to cold, and the deaths from consumption are numerous, even amongst the inhabitants. The climate of Italy, notwithstanding it has been described as a heaven of loveliness, and however pleasant it may be to persons in good health, affords no immunity from pulmonary disease. Two of the best localities in the Italian Peninsula for the residence of pulmonary invalids, are Como and Venice. The summer climate of Como is beautifully adapted for pulmonary complaints. The transitions of temperature are more gentle here than at any other station in Italy.

The climate of Venice is exempt from those violent atmospheric perturbations which are the bane of the Neapolitan seaboard; while it possesses a certain mildness of character and equability often unknown in some of the southern parts of Italy. Genoa is one of the most unfavorable localities in Italy for pulmonary complaints. Florence is equally prejudicial. The climate of Pisa is far too relaxing, humid and murky to be beneficial in tuberculous diseases. The Roman climate, if mild, is sedative and depressing; and owing its mildness to malarious emanations cannot prove salutary, particularly in a malady characterized by depression of the vital forces. A warm, humid, relaxing atmosphere cannot be of benefit in pulmonary disease. Cool, dry, and still air, as a general thing, is of much greater benefit, especially to those born in temperate regions. The climate of Naples is the worst in Italy for persons affected with disease of the respiratory organs.

Certain portions of Spain are much more favorable to persons suffering from pulmonary troubles than Italy. The whole of the Mediterranean coast of Spain has a southerly aspect; and as a general rule, walls of lofty mountains, running parallel to the sea, form a protective barrier to the north. Between these mountains and the sea are strips of smiling country, with warm and genial air, cloudless skies, and rich and luxuriant vegetation. The summers on this coast would be too warm, but for the rest of the year no more delicious climate can be found in the world. In the central portions of Spain the air is dry and rare, and often agitated by winds. The variations in temperature are sudden and extreme, rendering this portion of Spain decidedly unfavorable to pulmonary invalids.

There is no place on the continent of Europe possessing

a climate at once so mild and equable, with so little variation, as *Malaga*. Situated in the 36° 43′ of latitude, it is far to the south of any portion of the Italian Peninsula, and even of Sicily and Greece. A perpetual spring, connecting the autumn of one year with the summer of the next, exists throughout the year, during which vegetation proceeds unchecked. The natives spend a large portion of their time and seek their amusements in the open air; whilst many of the poor, the whole year through, care for no other beds than such as they can spread after nightfall upon the public walks.

The mean annual temperature of Malaga is 66·11°. The mean winter temperature 54·41°, being seven degrees warmer than Rome, seven than Nice, and eight than Pisa. The spring temperature is 62·55°, and the summer and autumn 79·38° and 68·67°, respectively. Thus it will be seen, the yearly range of temperature is only 49°, while in our climate there is as much variation in as many hours.

The mean daily range of temperature amounts to only 4·1°, and the mean difference between the temperature of successive months in winter is only 2·16°. Sometimes for twenty days the thermometer does not vary one degree, and when it varies the most it is so slight and gradual as to produce no unpleasant effects. As a winter residence for persons in the early stage of pulmonary difficulties, Malaga is undoubtedly one of the most favorable locations in the world.

If a more bracing atmosphere than Malaga is required, it will be found about two leagues from the city, in the village of Torre Molinos, the climate of which possesses a more tonic quality. A pleasant summer residence may be found at Fonda, about eleven leagues from Malaga, and more than four thousand feet above the level of the sea. Almeira, on the shore of the Mediterranean, possesses an extremely mild winter climate. Frost and snow are unknown, and the temperature rarely falls below 50°. The climate is one of the most healthy in Spain. The skies are clear and brilliant, and rarely obscured by clouds. Rain is of short duration, and the air is dry, light, and calm.

The climate of Algiers by some is considered even better than Malaga. It is certainly mild and healthy, and well adapted for chest complaints both of the heart and lungs. The latitude of Algiers is 36° 40′. The mean annual temperature is 64°. The temperature of spring is 60·5°, of summer 74°, of autumn 68°, and of winter 54°.

In summer, the upper current of air, which is in fact the Simoon or Sirocco, occasionally descends to the surface in Algeria. The effect of this wind upon human health and vegetation is pernicious. No invalid should remain during the season of this pestilential blast. Not only does pulmonary consumption, in Algeria, march with a slowness which gives nature time to organize her means of defence, and therefore of cure; but further, in modifying the constitution, it causes the latter to lose its tuberculous susceptibility. A case of consumption is very rarely met with among the old inhabitants of Algeria.

This climate is also recommended for cases of chronic bronchitis, chronic diseases of the heart, gout and rheumatism.

The Island of Madeira possesses a highly favorable climate for consumptive invalids. The weather is not subject to those extremes of heat and cold which are so trying to the invalid. During the summer the almost constant prevalence of northeasterly winds, especially on the north, and the regular sea and land breezes on the south side of the island, maintain the atmosphere in a temperate state. The sirocco, which occurs two or three times, at most, during the season, and then continues but two or three days, sometimes raises the thermometer in the shade to 90°. With this exception the summer temperature is very uniform, the thermometer seldom rising above 80°. In consequence of the regular sea-breezes, the heat is not oppressive. Close, sultry days are but little known, and there is neither smoke nor dust to impair the purity of the atmosphere. A distinguished physician, himself an invalid, who had resided some time on the island, said he thought the summer climate of Madeira quite as favorable to consumptive invalids as the winter.

The rainy season commences about the beginning of October, and is accompanied with westerly and southwesterly winds. In November the weather clears up, and generally continues fine and mild till the end of December. During January and February the weather continues more or less damp, but fog is never seen, and the thermometer at sunrise is seldom found below 50°. Patients intending to spend the winter in Madeira, should leave this country early in October, and returning, reach home about June.

The Bermudas, notwithstanding their variable climate, are undoubtedly much more healthy as a winter residence for a consumptive invalid, than the northeastern portion of the United States. The season from October to May is the most healthy, and the only part of the year during which this climate is at all suited to invalids. The climate is variable and windy during the winter, and hot and oppressive during the summer. There are, however, many beautiful spots in these islands, where, protected from the northerly gales by the cedar-clothed hills, the invalid might find sufficient space to exercise in the open air almost every day during the winter. The vicinity of the little town of Hamilton, nearly in the center of the islands, affords, perhaps, the most favorable situation for such a residence.

The West Indies.—The mean annual temperature of the West India Islands, near the sea, is about 79° or 80°. The temperature in winter is about 76° ; spring, 79° ; summer, 81° ; autumn, 80°. The extreme annual range does not amount to more than 15° or 20°. The winter and early part of the spring are dry and the weather fine ; the summer is dry and hot. Invalids should reach the West Indies about the first of December, and leave the last of April.

For confirmed consumption, the climate of these islands is not generally favorable, but in the incipient stage, a winter residence here may be highly beneficial, especially if the constitution is free from much disorder of the nervous system and digestive organs. In those cases where consumption depends chiefly upon hereditary predisposition, and occurs in early life, especially in feeble, irritable constitutions, this climate will rarely agree. Persons predisposed to bilious or stomach difficulties, should not go to the West Indies. In scrofulous diseases the climate is very favorable.

Among the most healthy islands in the West Indies, we may mention Jamaica, Barbadoes, St. Vincents, Antigua, and St. Christophers.

Jamaica.—In the mountainous districts of St. Andrew and Port Royal, there are residences and settlements three or four thousand feet above the level of the sea, where the air is cool and salubrious the year through. Probably the most healthy district in Jamaica is the mountainous part of the Parish of St. Ann, which is nearly in the centre of the island. The mean temperature of the year at this place is 76°. The climate of Lucea is also cool and pleasant, except during July, August, and September.

Barbadoes is comparatively level, but is one of the most healthy of the islands. Speightstown, on the northwest extremity of the island, is one of the best places for a town residence. The part of the island called Scotland is from 600 to 800 feet above the level of the sea, and receives the constant benefit of the trade winds. It is cooler than the lower part of the island, and is remarkably healthy.

St. Vincent lies directly to the west of Barbadoes. Its capital, Kingston, occupies a healthy situation on the shores of a fine bay. More cool and healthy situations may be found, however, by ascending the mountains which compose the greater bulk of this charming and romantic island.

St. Christophers (or St. Kitts) is one of the most lovely and healthy of all the West India islands. From its mountainous character, the invalid can have the advantage of a change of climate in the same island. It also has the advantage of excellent roads. It occupies a central position among a group of islands, among which the patient can cruise, making short visits to each with more advantage than by remaining all the time on one island.

AMERICAN CLIMATE.

As good a climate, with the exception, perhaps, of Malaga and Madeira, for any class of invalids can be found within the limits of our own country as in any portion of the world. The Peninsula of Florida possesses a peculiar climate, and there are places here which, for a winter's residence, cannot be surpassed by any place in the world. Jacksonville, situated on Tampa Bay, is a delightful spot for a winter's residence. The mild and equable temperature, the soft and balmy breezes of an ever-green land, renders the climate peculiarly grateful to those who have shivered in the rough winds and the ever-changing temperature of the north. St. Augustine is also a favorable location, although liable to more changes of temperature than Jacksonville and some other localities. The frequency and severity of the winds at St. Augustine constitute a considerable drawback on the benefit of the climate. The mean winter temperature at Tampa Bay is 64·76° ; at St. Augustine, 62·21°.

The climate in Florida is so mild and uniform that, beside the vegetable productions of the Southern States generally, many of a tropical character are produced. The lime, the orange, and the fig, find here a genial temperature. The course of vegetation is unceasing, and wild flowers spring up and flourish in the month of January. So little is the temperature of the lakes and rivers diminished, that one may bathe at any time in their waters.

Savannah possesses many advantages over our northern climate as a winter's residence. The climate is mild, although far less equable and salubrious than Florida.

Aikin, situated in the Southern portion of S. Carolina has advantages which many physicans esteem highly. It is located in the midst of immense pine forests, and in addition to its mild climate, the medicinal influence of these vast pineries in pulmonary complaints is highly beneficial.

As a summer residence, the vicinity of Lake Superior, portions of Wisconsin, Minnesota, and Kansas, are among the best in this country. The air has a peculiar bracing effect, highly beneficial to the weak and debilitated. A summer tour to Lake Superior, and over the wild prairies of the West, would, to many an invalid or care-worn man of business, be productive of far more good than a voyage across the Atlantic, and a hasty sojourn in the capitals of Europe. To the inhabitants of the West, a change to our ocean-washed shores, and the luxurious sea-bathing for the summer months, would invigorate the system, and bring back the hue of health to the faded cheek of many an invalid.

But those of us who live at the East and the South, will find amid the wild scenery of New England, the upper portion of New York, and in Western Virginia and Pennsylvania, in the vicinity of the Blue Ridge and the Alleghany mountains, many a cool nook and quiet resting-place, where, free from excessive summer heat, the invalid, living amid the grand and beautiful in nature, can recruit the wasted frame, and breathe new life in the pure and bracing air which eddies around the mountains, and gathers fragrance from the meadows and the forests.

The climate on the Pacific coast of the United States is much more mild and equable than on the eastern or Atlantic coast in the same latitude. Winter on the

Columbia River, in Oregon, is remarkablymild, the river being obstructed by ice only a few days in January. Grass remains, as a general thing, in sufficient perfection to afford good food throughout the winter. During a year's observation at Fort Vancouver, the lowest point of the thermometer was 17°, and the whole number of days below the freezing point were only nine, all of which were in January.

As we go still further south, to the golden State of California, we find not alone mines of glittering gold, but, especially in the southern and interior portions, a soil as rich as sun ever shone upon, and a climate as genial and as healthy as any in the world. Invalids might find the climate of San Francisco somewhat trying, on account of the occasional heavy northwest winds, but back in the interior, and in the southern portion of the State, localities may be found unsurpassed for beauty or healthfulness. In the middle of January, the air is as soft and balmy as in New England in June. True, among the mountains far back in the interior, the weather is at times intensely cold, but these are localities which the invalid would scarcely choose as a permanent residence.

To persons of weakly constitutions, predisposed to consumption, lacking nervous force, or whose systems are vitiated by scrofula, those growing States on the Pacific offer peculiar inducements. In that genial climate, the system may recruit, and become robust and strong, while here it might speedily languish and wither.

There is one other point in the Pacific to which I must

briefly refer. I mean that group of islands, now an isolated kingdom, washed on all sides by the waters of the Pacific, yet destined soon to take its place in our glorious confederacy of States—the Sandwich or Hawaiian Islands. The climate in these islands is delightful. The seasons glide imperceptibly into each other, and in the middle of winter the air is so soft and balmy that the inhabitants could almost live out of doors. The variations of the thermometer are very slight, the summers being comparatively cool. For the consumptive, or worn out and debilitated, a short residence here will frequently work an almost miraculous change. For almost any disease I would much prefer advising a voyage to the Pacific, and a short residence either in California or the Sandwich Islands, to a trip up the Mediterranean.

MINERAL WATERS.

The diseases most benefited by mineral waters are generally those which have had their origin in derangements of the digestive organs. The diseases of the skin, of the joints and nervous system, can usually be traced to some disturbance in the digestive apparatus. Among the most celebrated springs in Europe for bronchial diseases we may mention *Ems*, on the Rhine; *Bonnes* and *Cauterets*, among the Pyrenees; and *Mont D'Or*, in Auvergne. The Ems waters are mild, and deserve the preference where there is much general delicacy of constitution.

In gout, the waters of *Ems*, of *Carlsbad*, of *Marienbad*, of *Aix-la-Chapelle* and of *Wiesbaden*, often prove highly beneficial. The most obstinate forms of chronic rheumatism are often relieved by the baths of *Aix* in Saxony, or of *Cauterets* and *Baynnes-de-Suchon* among the Pyrenees, and those of *Aix-la-Chapelle.*

The sulphurous waters are often highly beneficial in scrofula and in chest difficulties, especially when complicated with derangement of the liver. In dyspepsia, rheumatism, gout and eruptive diseases, their use is often attended with the most happy results. These waters, however, should be used with care, and always omitted when they produce headache, a white tongue and some degree of febrile irritation. In the advanced stages of consumption, and especially in those predisposed to hemorrhage, the sulphurous waters, if used at all, should be very weak.

Among the celebrated waters of this class, are those of Aix-la-Chapelle, in a city of the same name, about thirty-six miles west of Cologne. Situated in the midst of a fertile valley, surrounded by high mountains, the air, a greater portion of the time, is salubrious and healthy. These springs were known to the Romans, but owe their modern fame to Charlemagne, who often held his levee in the bath, with all his attendants. The temperature of the different springs is from 110° to 136°.

The White Sulphur Springs, situated in Greenbriar county, Virginia, are deservedly celebrated throughout the country. The water is very cold, deposits sulphur in large quantities, and contains an abundance of saline substances. These springs have been found highly beneficial in chronic rheumatism, cutaneous diseases, and in the general prostration which sometimes follow remittent, bilious, or intermittent fevers. The Salt Sulphur and the Red Sulphur Springs in Virginia, are largely resorted to by invalids. The Red Sulphur is peculiarly adapted to affections of the chest, especially to pulmonary consumption. In addition to these springs, we may also mention as beneficial in the classes of diseases to which we have referred in speaking of these waters, several sulphurous springs in Kentucky and Tennessee, among which are the Big Bone Springs and the Olympian Springs; also the Sharon and Avon Springs in New York, which are frequented by large numbers of invalid

The Acidulous Waters deserve a brief mention. They contain carbonic acid in various proportions, and several salts, among which are muriate of soda, carbonate of lime, and sulphate and carbonate of iron. These waters are slightly tonic, allaying febrile irritation, stimulating the action of the liver, the stomach and the bowels, and invigorating the whole system. The Sweet Springs in Monroe county, Virginia, are the most celebrated of any of these waters, and have become a fashionable place of resort. Their temperature is 73°. The waters at Bath, Berkeley county, Virginia, nearly resemble the Sweet Springs.

The most celebrated acidulous springs in France are those of *Mont D'Or* and *Nichi*. At Mont D'Or, there are four baths. Three have a high temperature—107°, 109°, and 113°. The fourth is only 52°.

Chalybeate Mineral Waters.—These waters owe their characteristic properties to an impregnation of iron ; the oxide of iron being usually held dissolved by carbonic acid. They also contain several salts. These waters possess a decided tonic power, and in persons exhausted by disease, and whose chief complaint is languor, with cool skin, and pale, and moist tongue, they have an admirable effect. The most noted of these springs in Europe are Spa, in Belgium ; Pyrmont, in Westphalia ; Passy, near Paris ; and Tunbridge and Brighton, in England.

The Balston Springs, in New York, are perhaps the purest form of Chalybeate waters which can be found. The Bedford Springs, in Pennsylvania, are situated in the midst of a beautiful country, and the invalid not only has the advantage of the waters, but of some of the most charming scenery in the world. The Yellow Springs, the Brandywine, the Frankfort, the Hopkinton, and numerous other springs, during the proper months, are thronged with visitors. The Schooley's Mountain Springs are much visited by persons from New York. The water is extremely cold, the air cool and bracing, and the scenery grand and beautiful. Among the most noted of these springs in the West, are the Yellow Springs, in Greene county, Ohio.

The Saline Mineral Waters next claim a brief mention. The salts most usually present are the sulphates, muriates, and carbonates. These waters have a very decided action upon the liver, stomach and intestinal canal, and, through them, on other portions of the system. Affections of the head, chest, skin, and joints are often materially relieved, as well as troubles of the stomach and bowels.

Among the springs of this class in Europe, we may mention the *Carlsbad Waters*, in Bohemia. The principal spring has a temperature of 165°. These waters are celebrated in dyspeptic difficulties, as well as troubles of the kidneys and bladder. They should, of course, be avoided in apoplectic persons, or where there is danger of hemorrhage. The *Cheltenham Springs* are among the most famous in England. The *Seidlitz Waters*, in Bohemia, nine miles from Prague, have a great celebrity. Of the mineral springs of the United States, those of Saratoga, in New York, are by far the most celebrated. They cannot strictly be classed among the saline springs, but partake somewhat of the character of the acidulous and the chalybeates, containing both carbonic acid and iron. There are several springs here, but the Congress is the most celebrated. These waters have been celebrated in cases of dyspepsia, constipation of the bowels, and troubles of the kidneys and bladder ; also in chronic rheumatism, cutaneous eruptions, scrofula, chlorosis, and general prostration and debility. In consumption and acute diseases of the chest, these waters are generally injurious. One great benefit arising from a visit to these springs may be traced to the pleasant rides in the vicinity, and the company which throng there during the summer months. An invalid may be retired if he chooses; notwithstanding, he will have plenty of opportunities for dissipation.

Of the numerous other mineral springs in the United States we have not space to speak. The Warm Springs of Virginia and Carolina, and the saline springs of Kentucky and Tennesse, are justly celebrated. But at any of these springs change of air, pleasant company and judicious exercise in the open air, are highly important auxiliaries in the work of cure.

HINTS TO TRAVELERS.

Men are by far too apt, when away from the restraints of home, and the observing eyes of friends, to fall into careless habits. What matters a little indiscretion among strangers, or a slight disobedience, here and there, of moral or physical laws. And so a hundred little things are done or neglected without thought of the consequences. But, by and by, the truth forces itself on the mind, that nature cannot be cheated, and it matters but little to her whether her laws are violated in public or private, at home or among strangers—the effect upon the individual is alike the same.

The traveler should pay particular attention to his dress. This, of course, should be regulated according to climate; but, at all seasons of the year, and in all climates, flannel should be worn next the skin. This precaution is of as much importance in warm climates as in cold, in summer as in winter, as it guards the system materially against changes of temperature. In warm weather, the clothes should be frequently changed, and the body sponged with water. In cold or changeable climates, the body should be well protected, warm and dry.

In traveling from one part of the country to another, the traveler will experience, perhaps, more trouble from change of diet, and the peculiarities of water, than from almost any other source. The diet should be plain, simple, and nourishing, if it can be had. In dining at popular hotels, there is no necessity of eating at railroad speed through the whole bill-of-fare, or drinking all the wine and brandy in the decanters. It is true, a person cannot always eat a sufficient dinner in the five or ten minutes which are usually set apart in railroad time-tables, at certain hours of the day, for filling passengers' stomachs; but if he takes a glass of cold water instead of a cup of hot coffee, there will be no danger of burning his mouth, and if he devotes himself deliberately and industriously for a few moments to the mastication of substantial food, and if he has not time to finish, takes a sufficient quantity into the car with him, where he can finish his dinner in peace and quietness, he will feel much more comfortable than he would have done if he had forced down his dinner unmasticated, or gone without.

Change of water, especially on going into districts where the water is hard, impregnated with lime, is liable to produce derangement of the stomach and bowels, causing violent diarrhœa and dysentery. At first, the water should be drank sparingly, using freely, if they can be obtained, fruits and milk. In some of the wine-growing countries of Europe, the water is so bad that some of the pure light wines are used as a daily drink by all classes.

In travelling on business, it is, of course, impossible to be as particular as when at home, yet even among this class of persons, ordinary care will enable them to avoid many a pain, and preserve their health unimpaired.

The invalid, sojourning for a time in a foreign country, will find temperate habits, pleasant society and free exercise in the open air at proper times, important auxiliaries in the work of cure, without which, the purest, softest air, and the brightest sky, will often prove unavailing.

PART II.

TREATMENT OF DISEASE.

CHAPTER I.

DIAGNOSIS OF DISEASE.

In prescribing for varied forms of disease, it will be well to bear in mind the peculiarity of constitution and temperament, to ascertain, if possible, the cause of the difficulty, and to note with care those general symptoms, such as the condition of the pulse and urine, which will often give a correct idea of the extent and severity of the disease.

Constitution and Temperament.—A *plethoric constitution* is characterized by a florid complexion, frame full and robust, activity and strengh of body, and a strong, full pulse. There is a predisposition to local or general congestion.

A *feeble constitution* is directly the opposite of the foregoing. There is a deficiency in the generation of natural heat, and a tendency to become fatigued from slight exertion. The pulse is feeble and soft.

A *bilious constitution* is recognized by a dark or yellow skin, by a predisposition to derangement and irregularities of the digestive functions, and a tendency to constipation, &c.

An *apoplectic constitution*, may be known by the large head, almost buried beneath the shoulders, short, thick neck, thick-set frame, slow, full pulse, and tendency of blood to the brain.

A *nervous constitution*, is characterized by extreme sensitiveness and excitability of body and mind. The pulse is variable, quickly changing from rapid to slow. The person is liable to nervous disorders, and those spasmodic affections, which are not readily referable to any direct cause.

A *lymphatic*, or *mucus constitution*, may be recognized by the light complexion, the frame full and rounded, but the flesh soft and flaccid, and the muscular fibre yielding and relaxed. The circulation is sluggish, the pulse slow, the generation of heat deficient, and there is also a sensitiveness to cold. The patient is subject to slow and sluggish affections to catarrhal diseases, abscesses, accumulation of water about various organs. Acute diseases are liable to assume a chronic form, and run a slow and tedious course.

The *consumptive constitution* may be known by the clear, transparent skin, often with a bright spot on the cheek, flatness of the chest, slender and fragile form, long and spare neck, quick and small pulse, long, slender fingers, with large joints. The patient is peculiarly liable to affections of the lungs.

The Pulse.—In feeling the pulse, the fingers may be placed on the wrist, directly back of the root of the thumb and the joint of the wrist, and just within the external bone of the arm. Note particularly, not only its rapidity but also its peculiarities ; whether it is intermittent, hard, and wiry, or soft, feeble, and almost imperceptible. The beat of the healthy pulse depends much upon age, sex, temperament, and constitution.

In the adult male, of medium size, it generally numbers from 70 to 80 beats in a minute, while in the female it is more rapid, varying from 75 to 85 in a minute. From the age of fourteen to twenty, it is usually from 80 to 90 beats in a minute.

After a man has reached the prime of life, and enters on the declining scale, which in our climate usually occurs between the ages of 50 and 60, the frequency of the pulse is diminished, until, in old age, it may only number from 55 to 65 beats in a minute. I have given the usual standard of the pulse, in health, in the various stages of life, but cases are by no means rare, where, in perfect health, it may be much lower or higher than I have stated. If, however, the skin is moist, and at a natural heat, this would be no indication of disease. The pulse also may vary before or after a meal, and be excited or depressed from exercise or mental emotion. We should, of course, be cautious in attributing this temporary change to the influence of disease.

The Pulse in Disease.—The *rapid,* or *accelerated pulse,* is indicative of inflammation or fever, especially if strong, full, and hard ; if small and very rapid, it indicates a low state of debility, such as is often present in the latter stage of typhoid fever.

The *slow pulse*, if not habitual, may indicate debility or tendency of blood to the head, or, especially if full and strong, pressure on the brain. It is also generally found in old age.

The *hard* or *wiry* pulse is generally indicative of a high state of inflammation, although in old age it may be occasioned by a hardening of the arteries.

The *changeable* or *unequal* pulse denotes a derangement of the nervous system, and not unfrequently organic disease of the heart.

The *intermittent* pulse generally shows some trouble about the heart. It is sometimes, however, occasioned by intestinal affections.

The *full, strong* pulse indicates a full habit, while the weak pulse denotes a feeble state of the system.

The Urine.—Healthy urine should be of a brightish yellow or straw color, possessed of a slight ammoniacal smell, devoid of unpleasant odor, and precipating no sediment on standing. In old age, however, the urine may be slightly offensive, and darker in color than in early life. In persons leading an active life, the urine is of darker color than in those of sedentary habits; different varieties of food may also produce a sensible effect upon the color and smell of urine.

In fever, as the crisis declares itself, a sediment is perceptible. If the sediment is of a light or greyish color, and deposited shortly after emission, it is a favorable indication.

The red, or high-colored urine, if the pulse be accelerated, indicates the presence of fever. Urine of a saffron-color marks the presence of bile in the blood, and shows derangement of the liver; if it should be dark or black, it denotes a putrid state; if disturbed, heavy, muddy, or of a purple color, it shows a bad state of the system. If the urine is bloody or slimy, we may apprehend affections of the bladder or kidneys.

The Stools.—Constipation indicates a torpidity of the bowels; light stools show the absence of bile, and therefore a torpid condition of the liver; dark stools indicate a large secretion of bile. Relaxed stools indicate an inflammatory or irritated state of bowels, or when unattended with pain, paralysis of the intestines.

Nausea or Vomiting.—Habitual nausea and vomiting, without any apparent cause, shows a seated disease of the stomach. Throwing up food as soon as it is taken into the stomach, shows inflammation. If vomiting is preceded by a sense of fullness, or pain which is relieved by the act, it is usually occasioned by indigestion. If nausea or vomiting is accompanied by a severe pain in the head, it may be sympathetic with the brain; or with violent pain in the liver, the kidneys, or the bladder, it would indicate inflammation of these organs. Pain in the head is not unfrequently the result of a deranged state of the stomach.

Cough.—Cough may be produced by a direct irritation

of the lining membrane of the air-passages, or be sympathetic, arising from disturbance in some other organ.

A painful hacking cough, accompanied with some febrile symptoms, denotes inflammation of the lungs. A loud, hoarse cough points to the wind-pipe as the seat of difficulty. A deep, hollow cough usually accompanies tuberculous disease. A cough, attended with wheezing and difficulty of breathing, is indicative of asthma. A constant hacking, unattended with fever or pain, and accompanied with tickling in the throat, may be traced to a slight irritation of the throat or larynx

The Countenance.—A careful observer will often detect the character of disease from the appearance of the countenance.

A yellow or sallow countenance, indicates a derangement of the liver.

A red, flushed face indicates a rush of blood to the head ; while a pale, sickly countenance indicates a lack of vitality.

ADMINISTRATION OF REMEDIES.

The remedy should be selected with the utmost care, for to prescribe carelessly would not only do no good, but might result in positive harm. The symptoms should be closely compared with those delineated under the heads of that class of remedies most likely to be indicated. The cause of the disease has also an important bearing in the selection of the medicine. The mind should be directed to the leading symptoms, and while it is not necessary that *all* the symptoms noted should be present, yet the utmost care should be taken that there are no symptoms present not covered by the medicine.

The Dose and its Repetition.—The form of medicines used are tinctures, powders, dilutions and globules. For the sake of being more clearly understood, and for the convenience of the patient, we shall adopt, in this book, the globules. If, however, the tincture or powders are preferred by the intelligent laymen, two drops may be mixed in a glass half full of water, and a teaspoon given at a dose. Or, as much of the powder as can be placed on a five cent piece, may be put dry on the tongue.

Three of the globules may be placed dry on the tongue, or six of them may be mixed with six teaspoonfulls of pure cold water, and a teaspoonfull given at a dose. Pure water should be used, such as rain, or spring-water which has been boiled, and great care taken that the glass and spoon are perfectly clean. Both the glass and spoon should be thoroughly washed with cold water. If two medicines are to be given, the same spoon should not be used for both, unless it is washed after each dose. If the symptoms are evidently aggravated or made worse by the remedy, it is indicative that the medicine is too strong. In this case, one globule may be taken, or one teaspoonfull of the usual mixture again put into six teaspoonfulls, and a teaspoonfull of this given at a dose.

A medicinal aggravation may be readily distinguished from that occasioned by disease. The medicinal aggravation comes on suddenly, and without previous amelioration, while that occasioned by disease is more gradual in its progress, and generally follows an amelioration. In acute cases, the remedy may be given every hour, or two hours; while, in chronic affections, once or twice a day will generally be sufficient.

The medicine, if carefully selected, should receive a fair trial, and be continued so long as benefit results from its employment. In mild cases, one dose will often be sufficient to remove the disease. If in either, in acute or chronic diseases, an amelioration follows each administration, the intervals may be gradually increased. The medicine should not be taken within a half-hour of eating, either before or after a meal. Camphor or perfumery of all kinds should be avoided in the sick-room, as they have a tendency to antidote the remedy given, or complicate the symptoms of the disease.

RULES FOR DIET.

In the successful treatment of disease, much depends on the proper diet adopted by the patient during the period he is under the influence of the remedy. Not only should indigestible substances be avoided, but also those articles of food which are more or less medicinal in their character. By indulging in either, the remedy may be antidoted, or at least new symptoms developed, not at the time distinguishable from those produced by the disease, thus complicating the symptoms, and causing the loss of much valuable time.

Aliments Allowed.—Lemonade, or other mild acid drinks, water, pure or mixed with currant jelly, raspberry, or strawberry syrup ; and sometimes milk, or milk and water, cocoa, unspiced chocolate, arrow-root, farina, barley-water, rice-water, beef and mutton soup, mutton, beef, venison, and most kinds of game, soft boiled eggs, and fresh butter.

Occasionally *fish*, such as trout, cod, haddock, and fresh scale fish. Also oysters, unless, as along some part of the sea-shore, they are impregnated with copper.

Among vegetables, potatoes, green peas, cauliflower, spinach, mild turnips, parsnips, rice, and hominy.

Fruits, such as peaches, raspberries, strawberries, oranges, stewed or roasted apples, and pears ; also prunes, grapes, etc. They should be perfectly ripe and fresh.

Bread, light and not newly baked, and biscuit, free from soda or potash. Puddings, such as rice, arrow-root, sago, tapioca, maccaroni, vermicelli, etc. Salt and sugar should be used sparingly.

Aliments Prohibited.—Rich and highly-seasoned soups, such as turtle ; pork, veal, bacon, duck, goose, liver, and all varieties of salt meats and salt fish ; also smoked meat, smoked, potted, or pickled fish, eels, lobsters, crabs, and fish not having scales.

Cucumbers, celery, onions, garlic, radishes, parsley, horseradish, and asparagus ; also, all kinds of pickles, salads, and raw vegetables.

Pastry of all kinds, spices, aromatics, and artificial sauces, mustard, vinegar, cheese, confectionery, and almost the whole variety of nuts.

Diet plain, healthy, easy of digestion, should be adopted in all cases ; although, as I have already stated, different persons require, in the varied forms of disease and constitution, different varieties of food. Thus, in cases of diarrhœa, fruits and vegetables should be avoided, while a constipated state of the bowels requires a free use of these articles ; also when symptoms of fever are present, meat, butter, eggs, and other stimulating articles of food, should be avoided, confining the diet more particularly to fruits and farinaceous articles.

CHAPTER II.

DISEASES CONNECTED WITH THE RESPIRATORY ORGANS.

COLD.

IN the form of an ordinary cold, or influenza, a host of diseases gain a foothold in the system. If allowed to go on, as is often the case, from the reason that the first symptoms are so slight, they may gain such an ascendency as to bid defiance to human skill, or only be eradicated after long days of suffering.

Slight symptoms are very apt to be neglected, whereas, if they had been promptly met, long attacks of sickness might have been avoided. That trite old proverb should never be forgotten, "an ounce of prevention is worth a pound of cure."

The first effects of cold may show themselves in many different ways There may have been a sudden exposure to a cold draft of air, remaining for a considerable length of time with damp feet or damp clothes, or perhaps, owing to a sudden change of the weather, the clothing may be insufficient ; whatever is the cause, the pores of the skin are closed, the circulation disturbed, and either the whole system, or some organ in the body, is liable to be affected. The throat may become sore, the nose and air-passages of the lungs irritated, causing cough and sneezing; the bowels or urinary organs may be affected; rheumatic pains may dart through the muscles, or erysipelatous inflammation be developed on the surface; a cold shivering sensation, severe pain in the head, or an aching, bruised sensation in the muscles and bones, may be felt more or less distinctly. Whatever may be the symptoms, it is very evident there is a disturbance in the circulation which should be promptly met.

Fortunately, the treatment in this early stage of a general cold is exceedingly simple. The great remedies are, as a general thing, *Aconite*, *Bryonia*, *Belladonna*, and *Rhus*.

Aconite is the main remedy, alternating it, in case there are shiverings, pains in the bones or aching of the flesh, or soreness and oppression of the chest, with *Bryonia*, one hour apart.

If there should be violent pain in the head, or soreness of the throat, belladonna could be alternated with the aconite, one hour apart. Or, should there be rheumatic pains shooting through the system, or erysipelatous inflammation, *rhus* should be given in the same manner. Sometimes, however, the first symptoms of the cold are developed in the form of

GENERAL INFLUENZA, OR COLD IN THE HEAD.

This trouble very often seems to prevail as a kind of epidemic. At certain seasons of the year, when changes of temperature are frequent and sudden, it may affect to a greater or less extent, whole communities. For the sake of clearness, we shall notice two forms of influenza:

COLD IN THE HEAD, AND GENERAL INFLUENZA.

Cold in the head, usually commences with sneezing, watering of the eyes, sometimes with a burning, smarting sensation, and running or stoppage of the nose. These symptoms may be accompanied by shivering and feverish sensation, and pain, more or less severe, in the head, particularly over the eyes and about the root of the nose. If these symptoms are not checked, the irritation of the mucous membrane, which is now confined to the nose and passages leading back to the throat, may extent downward to the throat and chest, laying the foundation for serious troubles.

Treatment.—If taken promptly in the first stage, *camphor* will usually break up the irritation in a short time. But this remedy should be taken at the commencement; for if the trouble is allowed to become fully developed, the camphor will do but little good.

Dose.—One drop of the spirits of camphor (the saturated solution) may be given on a lump of sugar every hour until relief is obtained.

Arsenicum.—When the disease has passed its incipient stage, and become fully developed, it must be met by the appropriate remedy. Arsensicum is the remedy when there is an obstruction of the nose, and at the same time an acrid discharge producing a burning heat and excoriation of the nostrils ; or, when the nose is at one moment free and in a short time obstructed, the discharge being thin and burning. Feeling of general debility.

Dose.—Three globules dry on the tongue, or six in four table-spoonfuls of water, a table-spoonful at a dose. Give every two hours until relieved. If, however, the relief is but slight after the third dose has been taken, wait three hours, and then substitute *ipecac.*, administering it in the same manner.

Nux-vomica should be administered in the first stage, especially if there is dry obstruction during the night only, with confusion in the head and heaviness in the forehead ; running of the nose in the morning, with dryness in the night.

Dose.—Three globules every three hours until relieved, or until four doses have been taken, when, if no relief is obtained, wait two hours, and then select another remedy.

Mercurius.—This remedy is of great value where there is frequent sneezing, profuse watery discharge, redness, itching or aching pain, or pressing the nose ; pain in the limbs, restlessness, shivering, and feverish heat.

Dose.—Three globules every four hours, or six globules in three tea-spoons of water, a tea-spoon at the same intervals. If after three doses no amelioration is felt, wait two hours, and then give

Hepar Sulphuris.—This remedy is particlarly indicated when there is an aching sensation at the root of the nose and over the eyes ; also when cold air renews the difficulty, causing headache ; or there is a stoppage of only one nostril, and the pain in the head is aggravated by movement.

Dose.—Three globules every three hours, until relieved.

Belladonna should bo given if the pain is not relieved by hepar ; and especially should there be violent throbbing, pain, and a sensation of heat about the head.

Dose.—Three globules every two hours, or six globules in three tea-spoons of water—a tea-spoon at the same intervals.

Aconite will be found highly beneficial, especialy when there are indications of fever, such as heat or shivering, general restlessness, etc. It may be given either alone, or in alternation with some other remedy ; if alone, three globules should be given every two hours.

General Influenza, or General Cold.—In addition to the symptoms mentioned under Cold in the Head, there is more or less shivering, alternating with flashes of heat, violent headache, drowsiness, rheumatic pains, difficult breathing ; generally cough, more or less severe, and general debility. There is often pain in the back of the head, and sometimes a sensation as of water running down the back. All of these symptoms may, however, not be present.

In the commencement of the disease, *camphor* should be given, one drop every hour, until four doses have been given. If the difficulty is not ameliorated, some other appropriate remedy.

Aconite is always indicated where there is inflammatory

action, shown by a quick, hard, or full pulse, hot or dry skin, and sometimes short and hacking cough. When fever exists, especially in the early stage of the disease, aconite will prove invaluable. It may either be given alone, or in alternation with some other appropriate remedy.

Dose.—Six globules may be dissolved in four tea-spoons of water, a tea-spoon given every two hours.

Opium may be given in alternation with aconite, one hour apart, when there is stupor or great fullness about the head, and flushed face ; also when there is dry cough.

Belladonna is of great value when there is a dry, spasmodic cough, aggravated at night, and affecting the head ; hot, dry skin, sore throat, headache more or less severe, usually of a throbbing character, increased by moving, noise, or a light, increased pain on stooping or coughing. When these symptoms exist, in connection with high fever, it will be well to alternate the remedy with *Aconite.*

Dose.—Three globules on the tongue, or six globules in four tea-spoons of water ; a teaspoon every hour or two hours, according to the severity of the symptoms.

Mercurius.—Chillness, or alternate chills and heat, followed by perspiration, which does not however alleviate the sufferings ; acrid or watery discharge from the nose ; pains in the face and teeth ; red or watery eyes, sore throat, cough at first dry then moist, aching in the bones, and slimy diarrhea, with straining.

Dose.—Three globules on the tongue, or six dissolved

in four tea-spoons of water, a tea-spoonful every two hours. Should there be much soreness of the throat, together with some of the other symptoms enumerated under *Belladonna*, it would be well to alternate with that remedy one or two hours apart.

Bryonia is frequently of great benefit when there is violent aching, bursting pain in the front of the head; constant cough, accompanied with pain in the chest; shivering alternately with flushes of heat and a bruised sensation about the flesh.

Dose.—Three globules every two or three hours, according to the severity of the symptoms.

Rhus is indicated where there is great restlessness, especially at night, prostration, nightly cough and pains, relieved by change of position. Give the same as Bryonia.

Arsenicum.—Acrid corrosive discharge from the nose, shivering, with severe pains in the limbs, oppression of the chest, prostration of strength. Dry fatiguing cough, worse at night, sometimes with a sensation of dryness and burning in the throat.

Dose.—Three globules every two or three hours, according to the severity of the symptoms.

Nux-vomica.—Hoarse, hollow cough, excited by tickling in the throat, accompanied with headache, pain in the lower part of the back, constipation, obstruction of the nose, and sensation in the chest as of excoriation.

Dose.—Same as *Arsenicum.*

Diet and Regimen.—In the milder forms of cold but little change in the diet is necessary. During the inflammatory stage, highly-seasoned and stimulating food should be avoided, substituting fruits and light farinaceous food, easy of digestion.

Cloths wet with cold water should be applied to the head if the pain is violent; and if the throat is sore, a cloth wrung out in cold water placed around it, covering this with a dry bandage.

COUGH.

Cough may be occasioned by a slight irritation of the throat or air passages, or it may exist only as one of a group of symptoms, indicating a deep-seated disease of the lungs and throat, or it may be sympathetic, produced by a derangement of some important organ. The treatment of cough, when it is developed in connection with some important organ, is given in connection with those diseases in their appropriate place. When *cough* is the principal symptom, some of the following remedies will be indicated:

Aconite.—Violent short cough, with feverish heat and thirst; sometimes sense of constriction, or pain in the chest, and difficult breathing.

Dose.—Three globules, dry on the tongue, once in two hours.

Stibrum.—Dry, hollow, or hard cough; loose cough,

with rattling in the chest, rapid and difficult breathing, feverish sensation ; cough with nausea or vomiting. Give same as Aconite.

Ipecac.—Tickling or spasmodic cough, frequently accompanied by nausea and vomiting ; worse at night, or in cold air ; oppression of breathing, as if the lungs were filled with mucus.

Hepar-S.—Dry, hoarse, or deep cough, frequently excited by talking, stooping, or much exertion ; worse at night, and aggravated by exposure of any part of the body to the cold air.

Dose.—Three globules every three hours. (*See* Influenza.)

Phosphorus.—Cough excited by lying on the left side ; dry cough, from tickling in the throat ; hoarseness and pain in the chest, as from excoriation.

Dose.—Three globules every two or three hours. (*See* Preumonia.)

Carb.-v.—Dry, spasmodic cough, sometimes producing vomiting, aggravated by damp, cold weather, and worse in the morning ; or, towards evening, accompanied with a burning, excoriating pain in the chest.

Dose.—Three globules once in two hours.

Nux-vom.—Dry, hoarse, fatiguing, or spasmodic cough ; worse in the morning, and during the day. Oppression of the chest at night ; and, on lying down, with a feeling of heat and dryness in the mouth ; cough excited by tickling, scraping sensation, with feeling of roughness or rawness in the throat, accompanied with hoarseness, severe pain in the head, and a bruised sensation about the stomach.

Dose.—Three globules once in two or three hours.

Sulphur.—Particularly in obstinate cases, when the cough is dry, excited by food, or a deep inspiration, and worse at night. Cough, with expectoration of thick or fetid mucus or pus of a salt or sweetish taste:

Dose.—Three globules once in three hours.

Bryonia—Dry, catarrhal cough, particularly in the winter, and when produced by recent colds; frequently accompanied with shivering, followed by fever and rheumatic or aching pains in the head and limbs.

Dose.—Three globules on the tongue, or six dissolved in six tea-spoons of water; a tea-spoonful every two hours

Rhus.—Short, dry, nervous cough, excited by tickling in the chest, worse in the evening, and attended with restlessness and shortness of breath. Cough, with rheumatic pains in the side and chest, sometimes with expectoration of blood.

Dose.—Same as Bryonia.

Belladonna.—Violent spasmodic cough; dry, short, and hacking cough at night, renewed by the slightest movement; dry cough almost without intermission, day and night, with redness of the face, and sensation as if something were in the windpipe. Pains in the neck and head.

Dose.—Three globules every hour, until relieved.

Hyascramus.—The symptoms are similar to the above,

but more particularly indicated when the cough is worse on lying down, and is excited by a tickling in the throat. Give same as *Belladonna.*

Mercury.—Hoarse catarrhal cough, with watery discharge from the nose, or diarrhea. Dry cough worse towards evening, or at night, increased by talking, and sometimes attended with expectoration of blood.

Dose.—Three globules every three hours.

Dulcamara.—Loose cough after taking cold ; cough excited by taking a deep breath, worse when at rest. Give same as mercury.

Pulsatilla.—Severe shaking cough, worse at night, and frequently with retching and vomiting. Loose cough, with aching in the chest, hoarseness, cold in the head, and expectoration of bitter mucus.

Dose.—Three globules every two hours.

China.—Asthmatic cough at night, with pain in the cnest, or cough from ulceration of the lungs, or loss of blood. (*See* Consumption.)

Arsenicum.—Asthmatic cough and breathing; dry cough, worse at night, and sometimes with bloody expectoration, and a burning sensation over the body. (*See* Influenza and Asthma.)

Dose.—Three globules once in three hours.

HOARSENESS.

This is an affection of the upper portion of the windpipe, and frequently exists in connection with other diseases, such as measles, influenza, and severe disturbance about the chest and windpipe.

Pulsatilla.—May be given when there is almost complete extinction of the voice, loose cough, and discharge from the nose of thick, yellow mucus.

Dose.—Three globules on the tongue, or six in four teaspoons of water, a teaspoonful every four hours.

Mercurius.—Is particularly indicated when from the commencement there is a thin discharge from the nose; also when there is profuse perspiration, especially at night, a hoarse, rough voice, and a burning, tickling sensation in the throat. Give same as Pulsatilla. It may be given with benefit after that remedy.

Nux-vomica.—Hoarseness, worse in the morning, and accompanied with dry, rough, fatiguing cough.

Dose.—Three globules every three hours.

Sulphur.—Particularly in cold, damp weather; roughness and scraping in the throat; in obstinate or chronic cases when the voice is almost extinct.

Dose.—Three globules every four hours. It follows with benefit Pulsatilla or Mercurius.

Rhus.—When there is a sensation of rawness in the throat and chest, chilliness, pain in the limbs, hoarseness, worse after talking, difficult breathing, with sneezing and watery discharge from the nose.

Dose.—Three globules every three hours.

Hepar-S.—Hoarse cough, worse at night, and accompanied by a sensation of soreness in the throat and chest. Give every four hours.

Carb.-veg.—In chronic hoarseness, aggravated by talking, and worse in the morning, and also in wet weather.

Dose.—Three globules morning and evening.

Phosphorus.—Particularly indicated in chronic hoarseness, when there is a dryness in the throat and chest, sometimes with sensation of soreness, and voice almost extinct. Give same as *Carbo.*

Diet and Regimen.—The wet bandage, a cloth wrung out dry in cold water, placed around the throat, and a dry flannel over it, will materially aid the cure. After four or five doses have been taken, if no relief has been obtained, another remedy should be selected. The food should be plain, avoiding spices and wines.

PLEURISY.

The lungs, suspended within the walls of the chest, are covered with a smooth serous membrane, which is reflected back over the internal wall of the chest, thus forming a shut sack. This membrane in health secretes a watery fluid, which enables the lungs to rise and fall at each inspiration, one membrane gliding over the other without pain. But let this membrane become inflamed, and the watery secretion ceases, or changes its character. As the lung, in rising or falling at each inspiration, rubs against the opposite dry and inflamed membrane, the most intense pain is produced at every breath. This inflamed membrane may pour out from its diseased surface a large amount of watery fluid, coagulable lymph, pus, or blood. Thus the membrane, which invests the lungs, may by this coagulable lymph be firmly glued to the wall of the chest, or the lung may be compressed by the large amount of fluid secreted into the pleural cavity.

Symptoms.—After having been exposed to cold, a dampness or shivering sensation may be felt intermingled with flushes of heat. The patient then complains of severe lacerating pain in the side, which soon becomes short and stabbing, as if at each inspiration a sharp instrument were thrust into the chest, at a particular point. The breathing is short and hurried, the face flushed, the skin hot and dry, the pulse quick and feverish ; short, dry cough ; scanty and high-colored urine, general prostration and occasionally violent headache and delirium. Should much frothy mucus be expectorated, the disease is complicated with bronchitis ; should rust-colored sputa be brought up, the disease is complicated with pneumonia.

Treatment.—*Aconite* and *Bryonia* are the two prominent remedies in this disease. If the attack is violent the remedies may be given in alternation every half hour, gradually increasing the intervals to two hours, as the symptoms improve.

Dose.—Dissolve twelve globules of the remedy in six tea-spoons of water, giving a tea-spoonful at a dose.

Sulphur.—May follow the above remedies when the pain has been relieved. Three or four doses of three globules each, given at intervals of four hours, will usually complete the cure.

Mercurius.—May be required when, notwithstanding the fever has been subdued, the pain and shortness of breath still continue, and the patient is becoming exhausted by copious night sweats. Three globules may be given every three hours.

If during the night the patient should be restless and sleepless, one or two doses of *Belladonna* given at intervals of one hour, will quiet the system.

The above treatment will, as a general thing, control the most violent forms of pleurisy in a short time, without the aid of bleeding, leeching, blistering, and calomel, which in the allopathic school are considered so important in this disease.

Sometimes, from the commencement the disease is complicated with pneumonia or bronchitis, but even then the treatment is simple. (Consult also those diseases.)

Diet and Regimen.—Cold water or toast-water may be taken, but the diet during the febrile stage should be light, consisting of panada, toast, farina, or gruel, in addition to some of the cooling fruits, such as strawberries, raspberries, sweet apples, peaches, oranges, &c.

FALSE PLEURISY.

This disease is often mistaken for pleurisy, yet with a little care it can be very readily distinguished. It is a rheumatic affection of the muscles of the chest, and is usually preceded by pains in the neck and shoulders, and accompanied with but little, if any fever or thirst. The pain is often severe in the side, but the cough is slight.

Treatment.—Three globules of *Arnica* may be given every three hours. This, of itself, will often produce a cure; but if no relief is obtained after three doses have been taken, it may be alternated with Pulsatilla, two hours apart.

Bryonia.—When the pains are sharp, and cutting exceedingly violent during inspiration. Give the same as *Arnica.*

Nux-Vomica.—Shooting pains, with great sensibility of the external parts of the chest to the touch aggravated by movement and by deep inspiration. Give the same as *Arnica.*

INFLAMMATION OF THE LUNGS.—PNEUMONIA.

Inflammation of the lungs is usually produced by sudden changes of temperature, or exposure to cold, damp winds. It generally commences with chilliness, followed by heat. The breath is quick and painful. There is pain in the chest on taking a long breath; dry and deep, or quick and hacking cough, excited by deep breathing or talking. The patient dislikes to talk, and generally prefers lying on the back. There is usually more or less fever, which is sometimes accompanied by great pain in the head, parched tongue, dry and hot skin, and excessive thirst. After a time the fever may assume an intermittent type, going off in the morning and coming on in the afternoon; or it may assume a typhoid character, accompanied with prostration and muttering delirium. (*See* Typhoid Fever.)

Treatment.—The prominent remedies are *Aconite, Stibium, Bryonia,* and *Phosphorus.*

Aconite.—Is indicated when there is considerable fever, quick pulse, and painful, oppressed respiration. Should the cough be hard and dry, or loose and rattling, *Stibium* would be better than *Aconite.*

Dose.—Six globules may be dissolved in four tea-spoons of water, and a tea-spoon given every hour

Bryonia.—Will usually be indicated in alternation with Aconite or Stibium, especially if the oppression or pain in the chest is aggravated by movement with constant desire to cough. The cough is usually loose, and the expectoration white or slimy, or of a bloody character. There are frequently pains about the limbs, and constipation.

Dose.—If in alternation with either of the above remedies, give one hour apart; if alone give every three hours.

Phosphorus.—May be given when there are severe sticking pains in the chest, excited or aggravated by breathing, or coughing, shortness of breath, dry cough, and rust-colored expectoration. This remedy can very well be alternated with *Bryonia*, or with *Belladonna*, if there should be violent pain in the head.

Dose.—Three globules once in two or three hours.

Should typhoid symptoms set in, characterized by extreme restlessness, delirium, and stupor, quick and irregular breathing, and great prostration, Phosphorus is still the remedy. Give every two hours, followed after three or four doses, if necessary, by Arsenic. (*See* also Typhoid Fever.)

Diet and Regimen.—The same as in pleurisy.

LARYNGITIS.

This disease is an inflammation of a portion of the windpipe, and unless speedily controled, often runs a quick and fatal course. It corresponds in the adult to croup in the child. There is a sore throat, accompanied with restlessness, and in a short time difficulty of swallowing and breathing. The act of inspiration is protracted and wheezing, as if the air were drawn through a narrow tube. The distress is in the vicinity of the bone in the middle of the throat, called Adam's apple. If there is cough, it is harsh and husky. The voice is hoarse, or scarcely perceptible; the face flushed, and the skin hot and dry. As the disease advances, the distress increases; the breathing becomes more and more difficult, there is a constant desire for air, and unless relieved, death by strangulation speedily ensues.

Treatment.—Apply externally the wet bandage.

Aconite.—Should commence the treatment, giving three globules every hour for three hours, until the fever subsides, or until other symptoms are developed.

Stibium.—May be prefered to *Aconite*, where the symptoms commence with severity; hoarseness, dry, harsh, and ringing cough, sometimes almost suffocative. Give as above.

Belladonna.—May be given where there are spasms in the throat, rendering it difficult to swallow liquids, and where the throat presents a swollen and inflamed appearance. It may be alternated with either of the above remedies, one hour apart.

Spongia.—Is indicated where the breathing is shrill, and there is severe pain in the upper part of the windpipe. There is also an increase of hoarseness and difficult articulation.

Dose.—This remedy may be alternated with *Hepar*, three globules one hour apart. Or, if the fever is violent, with *Aconite* or *Stibium*, at the same intervals. A physician should be obtained as speedily as possible.

BRONCHITIS.

An inflammation of the lining membrane of the air-tubes of the lungs is called Bronchitis. It may be either acute or chronic. The acute form often follows cold in the head, although it may commence in the bronchia. It usually commences with a feeling of roughness in the throat, which soon excites a frequent dry and hard cough. There may be hoarseness, difficulty of breathing, and a feeling of oppression about the upper part of the chest. There is more or less fever, pain in the limbs, and rapidity of the pulse. As the cough increases in severity, the expectoration is usually of a frothy character, sometimes streaked with blood. If the disease terminate unfavorably, the breathing becomes more and more difficult, and the patient is speedily prostrated; if favorably, the breathing becomes less difficult, and the fever gradually abates.

Treatment.—Aconite is the main remedy while fever exists. It is particularly indicated where there is hot, dry skin, hoarseness, short, dry and frequent cough, excited by tickling in the throat and chest, difficulty of breathing, thirst, and scanty expectoration. *Stibium* may be prefered where there is a rattling, or hard, dry cough.

Dose.—Six globules in four tea-spoonsfuls of water, a tea-spoonful every two hours.

Spongia and *Hepar.*—May be given after the fever has been in a measure subdued by *Aconite,* when there is hoarseness and burning, tickling in the wind-pipe, anxious-labored breathing, and hollow, dry, or hoarse cough.

Dose.—If in alternation, give three globules two hours apart.

Nux-Vomica.—Difficult breathing and tightness in the chest, particularly at night. Dry cough, worse towards morning; constipation.

Dose.—Three globules every three or four hours.

Bryonia.—Difficult breathing, with constant inclination to take a deep breath; breathing impeded by shootings in the chest. Give the same as *Nux-vomica.*

Phosphorus.—Is a prominent remedy, especially after

the inflammatory symptoms have been subdued by *Aconite*, if the respiration continue oppressed, and there is a heat, or sore, and shooting pains in the throat and chest, dry cough, excited by tickling, aggravated by talking, or laughing, and accompanied with expectoration of stringy mucus with saltish taste.

Dose.—Three globules every three hours. (*See Pneumonia.*) A few doses of *Sulphur* given at intervals of four hours after the prominent symptoms have subsided, will usually complete a cure.

Diet and Regimen.—The same as in *Pleurisy.*

For the treatment of chronic Bronchitis the appropriate remedy may be found under the head of cough.

HEMORRHAGE FROM THE LUNGS.

Hemorrhage from the nose, mouth, or throat, is often mistaken for hemorrhage from the lungs, thereby causing unnecessary alarm. Hemorrhage from the lungs may arise from congestion, or as in consumption, be produced by an ulcerated and weakened state of the lung. In the latter case, the blood is of a bright, red color. Hemorrhage from congestion of blood to the lungs may be occasioned by violent exertion, mechanical injury, or the inhaling of poisonous gases, or breathing an air filled by injurious dust, as metal-filings, or the dust from lime, or tobacco ; or it may be produced by rapid change of temperature, or the abuse of spirituous drinks. It is frequently occasioned by suppression of blood from other organs, and may follow the sudden disappearance of piles, and in ladies, the suppression of the menses.

Treatment.—Where the hemorrhage is severe, perfect rest in a half-recumbent posture is absolutely essential. The patient should not be permitted to speak, and no unnecessary noise or confusion allowed. In absence of other remedies, half a tea-spoonful of table-salt may be given with care, so as not to produce choking, in a little water, every ten minutes ; or five drops of sulphuric acid may be mixed with a tumbler of water, and a table-spoonful given until relieved.

Aconite.—Is usually indicated at the commencement of the difficulty. There is usually a sense of fullness and burning pain in the chest, palpitation of the heart, restlessness and anxiety. The blood is discharged at short intervals.

Dose.—Twelve globules in six tea-spoonfuls of water, a tea-spoonful given in severe cases every twenty or thirty minutes. Where the fullness about the chest and the expectoration is slight, give every three or four hours.

Ipecac.—If, after the violent symptoms have been subdued by *Aconite*, there should still remain a taste of blood in the mouth, or be present a slight, hacking cough, this remedy may be given, three globules once in two hours.

Belladonna.—Slight cough, produced by tickling in the chest, with aggravation of the hemorrhage, and sensation as if the chest were full of blood, with shooting pains, worse by movement.

Dose.—Prepare the same as *Aconite*, with which it may

often be alternated one hour apart. If given alone, take every two hours.

Arnica.—Particularly where the difficulty has been occasioned by mechanical injuries or exertion, and where with but slight exertion, black coagulated blood is discharged, accompanied with stitches, burning, contracted pain in the chest, palpitation of the heart, and debility; or where with a cough, excited by irritation under the breast-bone, there is a discharge of bright, red, frothy blood, sometimes mixed with streaks of mucus.

Dose.—Three drops in a glass half full of water, every one or two hours, according to symptoms.

China.—Where there is weakness occasioned by loss of blood, or violent, dry, and painful cough, with taste of blood in the mouth, and shivering with flushes of heat and bewilderment of the head.

Dose.—Three globules every three hours.

Opium.—Particularly in intemperate persons, or where the blood is of a thick or frothy character, and accompanied with trembling and anxious starts.

Dose.—Three globules every two hours.

Nux-Vomica.—When occasioned by cold, anger, or sudden suppression of hemorrhoidal discharge. Also in drunkards, after *Opium*, and where the cough is worse towards morning.

Dose.—Three globules every four hours.

CONGESTION OF THE CHEST.

There is a sensation of fullness about the chest, sometimes palpitation of the heart, and oppressed breathing.

Nux-Vomica—Will produce relief when the trouble is produced by sedentary mode of life, abuse of spirituous drinks, or continued mental exertion. Also where there is palpitation of the heart, oppressed breathing, with great restlessness, and sensation of tightness around the chest.

Aconite.—Heat, thirst, violent oppression, and palpitation of the heart.

Phosphorus.—Oppression, with fullness and tightness in the chest, and sensation of heat extending into the throat.

Mercury.—Oppression, with desire to take a long breath, burning in the chest, and cough with expectoration of blood.

Belladonna.—Palpitation of the heart, and fullness about the head, shortness of breath, short cough internal heat, and thirst.

Dose.—Twelve globules of the remedy indicated may be mixed with six tea-spoonsfuls of water, and a tea spoonful given every four or six hours. (*See* also *Hemorrhage from the lungs, Bronchitis, and Cough.*)

PULMONARY CONSUMPTION.

This insidious disease, which in our ever-changing clime

is constantly reaping a fearful harvest, is, as a general thing, hereditary, although it is sometimes the result of moisture, bad air and food, dissipation, imprudence in dress, changes of temperature, and also sometimes follows other diseases. It is often developed in the children of those who, for generations, have shown no traces of the disease. But in these cases, it will generally be found, there has been some violation of nature's laws, either in improper marriage, or prostrating vices. (*See* Chapter III., also pages 52 and 59.)

Symptoms.—The incipient stage of consumption *can be cured*, and even where it is hereditary. I am strongly inclined to believe that by means of proper physical, moral, and mental training, a proper education of the whole system in childhood, in very many cases at least, children may escape the doom of the parents. I say that consumption, in its incipient stages, may be cured, but beware how you allow it to fasten its fangs deep in the system, how you disregard the slight, hacking cough, the growing sensation of languor, the weakness of the chest, the increasing flush on the cheek, and those other symptoms which, perhaps, if taken at first may be easily removed.

The general symptoms of phthisis are cough, shortness of breath, expectoration, hæmoptysis, night-sweats, and wasting; hectic fever, hoarseness, or loss of voice, diarrhea, and various other symptoms, marking the different stages of the disease.

Cough is one of the earliest symptoms. It is, at first, generally slight and dry, occurring particularly on getting into the bed at night, on getting up in the morning, or after any unusual exertion. It soon becomes more troublesome, and is attended with more or less expectoration. Hæmoptysis, another symptom, is the expectoration of blood. This is a common symptom; but I have already spoken of it under a separate head. As the disease progresses, the patient is troubled with shortness of breath after but very little exertion, and particularly on going up-stairs, or ascending even a slight eminence.

Hectic fever gradually steals on. The patient may, in the evening, feel chilly, and at night flushed and hot, the skin, particularly the hands and feet, dry and burning, followed during sleep and towards morning by profuse and exhausting perspiration. This perspiration is generally more copious on the upper part of the body, the chest, and the head, and almost invariably comes on during sleep, the patient on awakening often finding himself drenched.

Diarrhea is another very common symptom; more frequently occurring during the latter part of the disease, and rapidly prostrating the strength of the patient. The voice, sometimes for months, is almost entirely extinct, the patient grows weaker and weaker, until at length he glides, almost without a struggle, into the arms of death. Or, perhaps, for a time, the unpleasant symptoms may abate, the strength begins to return, and brightening hope whispers to the soul promises of returning health, when the blow falls, and all is over. In tubercular consumption, the tubercles may exist for years, without disturbing the health. If by proper treatment they are not removed, they soften and produce ulceration. The rapid form of consumption, which is frequently seen among the young, and after debilitating diseases, is rightly called *galloping consumption*, for its course is short.

In tuberculous persons, syphilitic and eruptive diseases, there is often a transfer of the disease from external organs to the lungs, developing a consumption which speedily ends in death.

Treatment.—The treatment of this disease in all its stages covers so broad a field as to render it not only impossible but unnecessary to go into the particulars here, as the skill and care of a judicious physician are necessary in its treatment. For the appropriate remedies in the incipient stage, consult *Cough*, *Bronchitis*, and *Inflammation of the Lungs*, also *Change of Climate*, page 80.

Diet and Regimen.—Cleanliness, fresh air, and as even a temperature as possible, are, of course, essential. Often simply a change of air, going from a cold to a warmer, or more temperate climate, will be sufficient to arrest a disease which seemed almost hopeless. In selecting the food, the wishes and feelings of the patient should be consulted, taking care, however, that, while the food is as nourishing as may be, it is as little stimulating as possible.

ASTHMA.

This peculiarly painful disease is often, though by no means in all cases, hereditary. There is great difficulty in breathing, coming on in paroxysms, and accompanied with loud, wheezing respiration. The attack is usually preceded by loss of appetite, languor, drowsiness, oppression, and chillness. There is a feeling of constriction about the chest, an urgent desire for fresh air, and a loud, wheezing respiration. These symptoms often last for several hours, and then gradually subside.

Causes.—The disease may be hereditary or it may be occasioned by peculiar states of the atmosphere, irritating the surface of the air-passages, or by certain influences, which affect, in a peculiar way, the nervous system.

Treatment.—When asthma is occasioned by congestion of blood to the chest, *Aconite, Belladonna, Nux-Vomica, Phosphorus*, or *Cuprum*, may be consulted. (*See* Congestion of the chest.)

By flatulence, *Nux-Vomica* or *Sulphur*.

In consequence of moral emotions, *Ignatia* or *Nux-Vomica.*

From suppressed catarrh, *Arsenica*, or *Ipecac.*

In aged persons, *Opium*, *Camphor*, or *Arsenic.*

Ipecac.—Is a very valuable remedy. Its indications are short, dry cough, nausea, cold perspiration on the forehead, rapid and moaning respiration, or respiration short and obstructed, as from dust. Nocturnal paroxysms of suffocation, rattling in the chest from mucus, and great anguish.

Dose.—Six globules in three tea-spoonfuls of water; in violent cases, a tea-spoonful every half hour.

Bryonia.—May be given after the third dose of *Ipecac*, if that remedy have produced no relief, or if the following symptoms be present. Respiration obstructed, and increased by talking or movement, particularly at night, or towards morning; cough, with pressure or shooting pain in the chest, aggravated by movement. Anxious respiration, intermixed with deep inspirations.

Dose.—Give three globules every two hours.

Arsenic.—Is often indicated after *Ipecac*, and is a prominent remedy in chronic as well as acute asthma. Difficult breathing, and accumulation of thick mucus in the chest; painful constriction of the chest and lungs, especially in a warm room; suffocative fits, particularly at night, when in bed, with panting and wheezing respiration, great anguish, and cold respiration. Increase of symptoms during rough weather, and on change of temperature.

Dose.—In acute cases, give three globules every half-hour; where the symptoms are less violent, every four or six hours.

Nux-Vomica.—Especially indicated where *Arsenic* or *Ipecac* fails to produce relief, and where the constriction is in the lower part of the chest, even the clothing there producing a sensation of oppression; short cough, with difficult expectoration; congestion of the chest with heat, burning, and general uneasiness.

Dose.—The same as *Bryonia.* (*See* also *Congestion of the Chest.*)

Phosphorus.—Difficulty of breathing and oppression of the chest, especially in the evening, and during movement. Nocturnal attacks of suffocation, palpitation of the heart, short cough, shooting pains, and fullness in the chest.

Dose.—The same as Bryonia.

Stibium.—Difficulty of breathing, with suffocative cough and oppression of the chest, arising from the presence of mucus in the air-passages ; rattling of mucus in the chest.

Dose.—Three globules every hour.

Diet and Regimen.—Persons subject to the Asthma, should bathe the chest morning and night with cold water. When the paroxysms are exceedingly severe, they may often be relieved by strong coffee, tobacco, or stramonium smoke.

AFFECTIONS OF THE HEART.

Diseases of the heart are of such a character as to require the advice and care of a judicious physician. As it would be impossible to enter into the minutiæ of the variety of diseases which may affect this organ, we shall only give some few general remedies.

Where the palpitation of the heart is occasioned by congestion of blood to the chest, *Aconite*, *Belladonna*, *Nux-Vomica*, or *Phosphorus* may be given. (*See* also *Congestion of the Chest.*)

After moral emotion, *Ignatia* or *Nux-Vomica.*

After fright, *Opium.*

From disappointment, *Ignatia* or *Nux-Vomica.*

From fear or anguish, *Veratrum.*

From loss of blood, *China.*

Dose.—Three globules of the remedy indicated, may be given every one, four, or six hours, according to symptoms.

CHAPTER III.

FEVERS.

In perfect health every organ in the body should perform its proper amount of labor. The machinery of the whole system would then move in harmony, and without pain. But let any of the organs of the system be prevented from performing their duty, and the whole circulation is disturbed, and an extra amount of labor thrown upon other organs. The effort of nature to throw off those clogs which prevent its free action, and restore equilibrium in the system, gives rise to fever. This struggle, of course, causes an increased combustion, and a derangement of the circulation is the result.

Take, for instance, the skin, and let those pores through which such a vast amount of perspiration, the result of combustion within, is constantly passing off, be closed by a sudden current of air, or any other cause, and the whole economy of nature is at once disturbed. The combustion is constantly going on within, but the avenues by which impurities were formerly thrown from the system are closed, and the torturing pain, and burning skin, and rapid pulse, are the result. And thus any disturbance or inaction of the respiratory or digestive organs is attended by peculiar symptoms, and derangement of the vital forces. Nature, deranged in her movements, struggles manfully to vindicate her rights. But the disturbing cause may be too great for her unassisted strength, and she sinks paralyzed, or, roused into too violent action, a highly inflammatory state is the result. In both cases, without help, the end may be death.

Now is the time for human skill to step in and aid nature in her efforts for relief. To do this effectually, it certainly is not necessary to prostrate the system to the brink of the grave, but the more simple the remedy, and the more directly it can be applied to the diseased point, the more quick the cure, and the more easily does nature get back into her old tracks.

General Directions in Fever.—Absolute rest, both of mind and body, are essential. The food should be light in its character, and easy of digestion. Ice-water, or ice, held in the mouth, can be given in small quantities at a time, with perfect safety. Toast-water, or even lemonade, can also be given, save in looseness of the bowels, or while under the influence of aconite, when acids should be avoided. Should the fever be high, frequent ablutions in cold water are highly refreshing. The room should be well ventilated, and kept as nearly as possible at an even temperature, say from sixty to seventy degrees. The patient should be placed on a mattress, and the amount of covering regulated by his own feelings. The linen should be frequently changed. In nearly all cases, save when the bowels are disordered, fruits, but little if any tart, such as roast apples, oranges, strawberries, raspberries, and peaches.

SIMPLE FEVER.

This fever is generally the result of suppressed perspiration, sudden changes of temperature, or undue exposure to heat, or cold ; also of mental emotion, and derangement in living.

Symptoms.—A chill or shivering sensation, preceded by lassitude, and followed by heat, quick pulse, dry skin, and coated tongue. There is more or less aching in the limbs, heaviness in the head, which may pass into a severe pain in the forehead ; thirst, and restlessness. The symptoms are often worse in the evening, abating toward midnight. When not the forerunner of other diseases, it usually runs its course in a few days.

Treatment.—*Aconite* will almost always dissipate the symptoms, unless they are the precursor of some violent disease ; but even in this case *Aconite*, at this stage, is still the remedy.

Dose.—Dissolve six globules in a half a glass of water, and give a tea-spoonful every two hours, until the skin becomes moist.

INFLAMMATORY FEVER.

The cause and premonitory symptoms of this fever are similar to *simple fever*. The symptoms are, however, much more violent. The chill is of longer duration, the tongue is coated, or of a bright red appearance, the urine red and scanty, the skin dry and hot. It generally runs its course in seven or fourteen days. A diarrhea, profuse perspiration, or bleeding at the nose, are not uncommon indications of a speedy and favorable termination of the disease. It easily assumes a typhoid character, but this termination in homeopathic treatment can generally be avoided.

Treatment.—*Aconite* is the first remedy which should be given. The inflammatory state of the system clearly indicates its use.

Dose.—Twelve globules in a glass half-full of water, a tea-spoonful every two hours, until a moist skin, and decreased frequency of the pulse show an improvement.

Belladonna.—Should there be fullness and heat in the head, dizziness, throbbing pain, and great sensitiveness to noise or light. This remedy, prepared the same as Aconite, may be alternated with it one hour apart.

Bryonia.—Is indicated where there are shooting or aching pains in the limbs, violent, stupefying pain in the head, with dizziness on rising or moving; delirium, pressure at the pit of the stomach, constipation, thirst and burning, dry heat mingled with chills.

Dose.—Dissolve twelve globules in a glass half-full of water, and give a tea-spoonful every three hours, or, should much fever be present, alternate with Aconite one hour apart.

Diet and Regimen.—Cold water and fruits, but little

acid, may be given, but the food must be light in its character, such as toast, panada, or farina. When the fever subsides, bread and meat, in moderate quantities, may be sparingly used.

NERVOUS OR TYPHOID FEVER.

This is a low sinking fever, affecting particularly the nervous system. The *ship* and *hospital fevers* are varieties of this disease.

Causes.—Badly ventilated rooms, exposure, want of cleanliness, unhealthy food, and hunger, are among the causes for its development among the poor. It may also arise from grief, care, violent exertion of mind or body, prostration from disease, or from the prostrating effects of that kind of medical treatment which, with its heroic depletion is often worse than the disease itself. Dampness, cold, or a peculiar state of the atmosphere, failing to give sufficient sustenance to the vital forces, may develop epidemic Typhus.

Symptoms.—During the premonitory stage, or in a mild form of the disease, the patient is languid, easily tired, and loses his appetite. The tongue becomes white, and is inclined to tremble. Wandering pains are felt in the head, back, and extremities, together with fullness and giddiness in the head ; unrefreshing sleep. These symptoms may last for weeks.

The commencement of the fever is marked by slow chills, alternating with heat, and sometimes violent pain in the head or back. The skin is hot and dry, the tongue is variable, smooth, and red, or dry, or coated, with red edges, and a dark brown streak in the center. Delirium is frequently present, sometimes of violent character, but usually low and muttering, with a perfect indifference to everything. Stupor, gradual sinking down in the bed, and diarrhea, are among the symptoms which denote the progress of the disease. The disease not unfrequently continues twenty-one or twenty-eight days, although in mild cases its course is much shorter.

Treatment.—Quiet, cleanliness, a room well ventilated, are, of course, essential.

If during the precursory symptoms there should be lassitude, chillness, with alternate heat, headache, rheumatic pains, and restlessness at night, Bryonia and Rhus may be alternated, three globules three hours apart.

Aconite.—When at the commencement of epidemic typhus, inflammatory symptoms declare themselves, such as a dry, burning skin, hard and full pulse, heat in the head, and thirst.

Dose.—Six globules in a glass half-full of water, a teaspoonful once in two hours, until better, or some other remedy is more strongly indicated.

Belladonna.—Twitching of the limbs, and feeling of restlessness. Drowsiness; the countenance changing from red to pale, and from cold to hot. Headache, more or less violent; violent throbbing of the arteries of the head and neck; pressing pain in the temples, intolerance to noise; delirium, starts as from affright. The tongue red, burning hot, and parched, the mouth and throat dry.

Dose.—Six globules in six tea-spoonfuls of water, a tea-spoonful every two hours.

Bryonia.—Bruised, aching sensation throughout the whole body ; pressing pain in the forehead, particularly on moving or looking up ; burning heat in the head, while the forehead may be covered with a cold sweat; moaning during sleep, heat, and frightful dreams. Heat, alternating with chillness, bitter taste in the mouth, nausea, and constipation.

Dose.—Give the same as Belladonna.

Rhus.—When in the precursory stage there is chillness even near the fire ; bruised, stiff, or lame sensation when at rest, relieved by motion, and drawing, and rigidity in the nape of the neck and back. As the disease advances there is great weakness and prostration, restlessness at night, with anguish, or sleep with murmurs, snoring, dry heat, or disturbed by dreams and frequent starting. Talkative delirium, stupefying headache. Oppression of the chest, diarrhea, followed by pain in the limbs, and prostration. Rhus is frequently indicated, especially in the commencement of the disease, and when it has been produced by dampness, in alternation with Bryonia.

Dose.—Twelve globules in a glass half-full of water, a tea-spoonful, in severe cases, every two hours, when the symptoms are less violent, every four hours.

Opium.—Is indicated when there is a constant desire to sleep, with snoring respiration, and hard, full pulse. Give the same as Rhus.

Phosphorus.—Especially when caused by cold or venereal excess. In the commencement of the disease, rheumatic pain in the limbs, worse morning and evening, increased by cold air, or the touch, and sometimes accompanied with a general sensation of sickness, weary, and bruised sensation, palpitation of the heart. As the disease progresses there is a small, quick pulse, and profuse sweat; sleep interrupted by shrieks, moaning and rattling in the chest, oppressive cough, and bloody expectoration. The above symptoms in typhoid pneumonia clearly indicate this remedy.

Dose.—Twelve globules in six tea-spoonfuls of water, a tea-spoonful every three hours.

Arsenicum.—Rapid prostration of strength, deathly countenance, eyes dull and glassy, low, muttering delirium, dryness of the tongue, dry and burning skin, thirst, and diarrhea; pulse weak, or scarcely perceptible.

Dose.—Three globules every hour. Should the evacuations be fetid, and cold perspiration on the face and extremities,

Carbo.—May be given in alternation an hour apart.

Diet and Regimen.—The same as in fever. In the low-sinking stage, however, it may be necessary to support the strength by means of beef-tea, and brandy.

REMITTENT OR BILIOUS FEVER.

This fever is more violent in the Southern and Western States, particularly where the country is new, and the vegetation rich. In more temperate climates it is developed more particularly in the spring, or during the great heat of summer. It may be occasioned by indiscretion in diet, exposure to changes of temperature, and any of the numerous causes, by which the digestive organs are disturbed.

Symptoms—Among the premonitory symptoms are headache, general uneasiness, and a deranged state of the stomach. A chilly sensation is followed or intermingled with flushes of heat. The mouth is clammy and dry ; pain in the head, back, and limbs, dry skin, flushed face, full and rapid pulse, and sometimes delirium. The tongue is white, occasional vomiting ; urine high-colored, and bowels constipated. In twelve or fourteen hours a remission of the fever takes place, although the fever does not entirely subside. After a calm of two or three hours the exacerbation again takes place, becoming shorter in duration, and less violent as the disease abates. In the more severe forms of the disease this remission is scarcely perceptible, yet the gastric irritability and the symptoms above noted, clearly show the character of the disease.

Treatment.—*Aconite.* Fever, thirst, yellow-coating of the tongue ; bitter, greenish, or slimy vomiting, painfulness in the region of the stomach, and severe headache. It may be well to alternate with *Bryonia*, *Belladonna*, or *Pulsatilla*.

Dose.—Twelve globules in six tea-spoons of water, a tea-spoonful every two hours.

Bryonia.—Particularly when the fever occurs in hot weather, with a damp and sultry atmosphere. Aching or tired sensation in the head, back, and limbs ; insipid or bitter taste, especially on waking ; heat, or shivering, with heat in the face ; desire for acids, and aversion to food ; dry, brownish-yellow tongue ; bilious vomiting, especially after drinking.

Dose.—Twelve globules in a glass half-full of water, a tea-spoon every three hours.

Belladonna.—Throbbing and beating pain in the head, particularly the forehead, with feeling as if the head would burst. Pain in the head, aggravated by moving the eyes, by light, or noise. Heat about the head with thirst, alternating with chills ; vomiting of sour or bitter substances.

Dose.—If in alternation with Aconite, three globules one hour apart ; if alone, the same every two hours.

Stibium.—Often in alternation with Bryonia, especially when there is nausea, aching pain in the head, bruised sensation in the limbs, dry heat, and rapid pulse.

Dose.—Three globules every two hours.

Ipecac.—Especially in the first of the disease, when there is loathing of food, nausea, and vomiting. Fullness in the stomach ; diarrhea ; aching in the forehead.

Dose.—Three globules once in two hours, until the symptoms change.

Pulsatilla.—Flat, pappy or bitter taste, belching of wind ; desire for acids, nausea ; vomiting of sour and bitter substances ; inclination to diarrhea, and frequent shivering. Give same as Ipecac.

Veratrum.—Debility after a stool ; stool with cramp-like pain ; soreness of the abdomen to pressure ; bilious vomiting and diarrhea.

Dose.—Three globules every two hours.

Nux-Vomica.—Bitter taste, nausea, particularly in the open air ; pressure and fullness in the stomach, constipation, spasmodic colic. Ineffectual urging to stool, aching in the forehead with dizziness; bruised sensation in the limbs.

Dose.—In severe cases three globules may be given every three hours. When the symptoms are less severe, every six hours.

Mercurius.—Putrid or bitter taste, and vomiting of slimy or bitter substances. Painful tenderness in the pit of the stomach, and below the short ribs, particularly at night, with anguish or restlessness.

Dose.—The same as *Nux-Vomica.*

Diet and Regimen.—During the fever the diet should be light, consisting of toast, farina, panada, and such farinaceous articles of diet with, if no diarrhea is present, ripe fruits. As the fever subsides the diet may gradually become more nourishing, commencing with broth, and coming back by degrees to the original diet, taking care, however, not to overload the stomach.

INTERMITTENT FEVER.*

The symptoms of this fever are so marked that there is no difficulty in distinguishing it from all other forms. In

* A large portion of this article is taken from my work on "Domestic Practice."

Remittent Fever, the fever is never entirely absent during the remission, while in Intermittent the paroxysm comes on, and in a few hours passes entirely off, leaving the patient without any perceptible trace of the fever.

It prevails more extensively in marshy countries, particularly at the south and west, where the land is being drained, and the rich soil turned up by the plough. The air is poisoned with a miasm so subtle in its character as to defy detection, and yet so powerful as to prostrate the strongest man. This fever may also be developed after other diseases.

Symptoms.—The paroxysm is generally marked by three distinct stages, viz.: 1st, *cold;* 2d, *fever;* and 3rd, *sweating stage;* although these stages sometimes seem commingled together.

In some cases the paroxysms appear every day, in others every other day, and again, once in three or four days, or even one or two weeks apart.

The Cold Stage.—Is preceded by headache, languor, and a stretching sensation; blueness of the nails. The coldness and shivering of the limbs and back gradually increase, and pervade the whole body; the teeth chatter, the shivering is so violent as to shake the bed, and the application of external warmth produces no immediate effect. There is oppression of the chest, pain of the head, or stupor, and delirium.

This stage varies in violence and duration, lasting from half an hour to three hours, when it is followed by the *hot stage.*

This stage is characterized by violent fever, quick, wiry, and rapid pulse, great thirst, dry skin, flushed face, pain in the head, and sometimes delirium, hurried breathing, and sometimes oppression of the chest. It lasts from three to twelve hours, when it usually terminates in the sweating stage, or, as is sometimes the case, runs into Remittent or Continued Fever. Sometimes the sweating stage is entirely wanting.

Sweating Stage.—The violence of the fever begins to abate, and is succeeded by profuse perspiration; the pulse becomes less full, and the aches and pains rapidly disappear, until all traces of the former violent paroxysm have subsided.

Treatment.—A prominent remedy in distinctly marked Intermittent, where all three of the stages are clearly and distinctly defined, is undoubtedly *Quinine.* Those of our Allopathic friends, who denounce so bitterly Homeopathy, cure their patients by this drug, which always in this disease, when it acts beneficially, acts homeopathically.

Dose.—Ten grains may be mixed with twice that quantity of white sugar, and divided into ten parts, a powder of which can be taken every four hours, during the intermission of the paroxysm. During the paroxysm the remedy must be discontinued. If the paroxysms should not return, a powder should still be taken, an hour before the usual time of the paroxysm, until after the seventh day. The fourteenth and twenty-first day should also be noted, and if any lassitude or derangement of the system be apparent, a powder should be taken. The effects of this drug should be watched, and if it brings on intense headache, and violent oppression of the chest, it should be discontinued.

Ipecac.—Shivering with but little heat, or heat with but little shivering; shivering increased by external warmth; oppression of the stomach, nausea, and vomiting. This remedy is particularly indicated where the third or sweating stage is scarcely perceptible.

Dose.—Three globules should be given every three hours, between the paroxysms, and three globules of *Nux* immediately after the attack. During the hot stage twelve globules of *Aconite* may be mixed in a half glass of water, and a tea-spoonful given every hour until sweating commences.

Nux-Vomica.—Particularly where the bowels are constipated, and in those fevers where the paroxysm comes on every day, or every other day, generally in the afternoon, the evening, or night, and where there is aching pain in the forehead, dizziness, nausea, and bitter taste; spasms in the stomach, and great weakness. It is also useful where there is paralytic weakness of the limbs, and dizziness, difficult breathing, or violent headache, increased by walking in the open air.

Dose.—During the interval between the paroxysms three globules every three hours.

Arsenic.—Particularly indicated where the stages are not distinctly marked, but are in a measure commingled; or where there is burning heat, with anguish, restlessness, and great thirst; great prostration of strength, nausea, retching, and vomiting.

Dose.—During the intermission of the paroxysm, three globules every three hours.

Pulsatilla.—Where there is vomiting of mucus, moderate thirst, pain in the head, and oppression of the head during the cold stage, and shivering when uncovered, during the hot and sweating stage.

Dose.—Three globules every three hours during the intermission of the fever.

Bryonia.—Where the paroxysms are preceded by dizziness and pain in the forehead, coldness is more prominent than the heat. During the chilly and hot stage there may be dry cough, stinging in the chest, difficulty of breathing, and nausea.

Dose.—Three globules every three hours during the intermission of fever.

Belladonna.—When there is violent throbbing, pulsating headache, with redness of the face; three globules may be given every two hours during the fever.

Veratrum.—During the paroxysm general coldness with cold, clammy sweat, or internal heat; or where there is cutting colic with painful diarrhea.

Dose.—Three globules may be given every three hours during the intermission of the fever.

China.—Before the fever, nausea, headache, anxiety, palpitation of the heart. Shivering, alternating with heat, or heat long after the chill. Uneasy sleep, yellow complexion, and general gastric symptoms.

Dose.—Three globules every three hours during the intermission of the fever.

Diet and Regimen.—Care should be taken to avoid unnecessary exposure. On the days when there is no paroxysm the appetite may be moderately indulged.

YELLOW FEVER.

This disease is seldom known in temperate regions, but prevails sometimes to a fearful extent in warm countries, where it is looked upon with as much dread as the cholera.

Causes.—Animal and vegetable substances exposed to continued heat in a moist atmosphere, soon decay and fill the air with a poisonous miasm. This miasm may give rise to yellow fever, especially when it exists in populous cities, and in crowded and ill-ventilated rooms and cellars.

Other prominent causes are exposure to the intense heat of the sun at mid-day, mental anxiety, want of cleanliness, dissipation, and excesses both in food and drink.

It is exceedingly fatal among persons who are accustomed to northern climates, and indulge as freely in the warm atmosphere of the south in stimulating food and drink, as in the colder north. As a matter, of course, the food is not all digested, and derangement of the system is the result.

Symptoms.—This disease often runs its course with frightful rapidity, terminating even in a few hours in death. In other cases the disease is more slow in its progress, its severity depending much upon the constitution, habits and temperament of the patient. The first symptoms are generally want of appetite, constipation, oppression of the stomach, giddiness and debility. When the attack comes on with violence, there is shuddering, headache, nausea, and vomiting. This is followed by severe pain in the back, and tearing in the limbs, sometimes amounting to cramps. These sensations last for a few hours, and are followed by violent reaction. The breathing becomes difficult, the breath burning, the pulse hard, full, and quick, violent pain in the head and throughout the body; dry and hot skin, thirst, nausea, and vomiting. The abdomen is hard and painful, and there is great suffering in the stomach. This period, lasting from a few hours to three or four days, is followed by almost an entire remission of suffering; but this is shortly followed by the return of the old symptoms. The skin and eyes are of a yellow tinge. The tongue is parched and covered with a dark fur, the skin clammy, the head confused, the pulse sinks, delirium may set in, the stomach is painful and sensitive, and the matter vomited presents a thicker and darker appearance.

This stage lasts from twelve to forty-eight hours, when it is followed by the third stage, characterized by extreme prostration; the tongue and lips are parched and cracked, the gums soft and livid, exuding black blood; there is intense suffering in the stomach, great anxiety, the dreaded *black vomit* growing darker and darker, and more and more frequent, until death closes the painful scene. On the setting in of the third stage the patient is usually beyond hope.

Treatment.—It is in diseases like this, where the ground has to be contested inch by inch, that medical skill is tested, and here it is when other systems are confused and panic stricken, that homeopathy marches on victorious.

Ipecac.—Is indicated in the first stage when slight chills, general pains, uneasiness in the stomach, nausea, and vomiting, together with a sensation of faintness, are present.

Dose.—Three globules every two hours.

Aconite.—Is indicated where there is violent febrile reaction, dry and hot skin, great thirst, full and rapid pulse, short and anxious respiration, restlessness and anguish ; pain in the head, back, and limbs, and sensitiveness in the stomach ; nausea, vomiting, and a general sense of prostration.

Dose.—Twelve globules in six tea-spoonfuls of water, a tea-spoonful every hour or every two hours.

Belladonna.—Particularly in the first stage of the disease, where there are shooting or violent throbbing pains in the head ; eyes sparkling and red, or fixed glistening and prominent ; pulse variable ; aching and cramp-like pain in the loins, back and legs.

Dose.—It is often necessary to alternate with *Aconite*, one hour apart. When given alone, give every two hours.

Bryonia.—Headache, increased by movement ; pains in the back, loins, and limbs, yellow skin, eyes painful on motion, pain and burning in the stomach, or fullness and oppression, vomiting, or nausea, particularly after eating.

Dose.—Three globules every two hours.

Rhus.—Sunken eyes, dry and black tongue, quick and small pulse, talkative delirium, or partial stupor, moaning, and great restlessness, particularly at night. Violent pain and burning in the stomach, spasms in the abdomen, numbness, or partial paralysis of the lower extremities.

Dose.—Same as *Bryonia.*

Nux-Vomica—Eyes yellow and inflamed, yellow skin, dizziness, pains in the head, pressure, cramp-like, or burning pain in the stomach, bilious or acid vomiting, trembling of the limbs, movements of slimy, bloody, or bilious matter, numbness in the lower extremities.

Dose.—Three globules every two hours.

Mercurius.—Pulse changeable, feeling of fatigue, dizziness, convulsive vomiting of bilious matter, tenderness of the stomach, constipation, or loose mucus, bloody, or bilious discharges.

Dose.—Same as *Nux.*

Arsenic.—Changeable expression of countenance, sunken eyes, surrounded by a dark circle, lips and tongue brown or black, cold, clammy sweat, small, trembling, pulse, great prostration, burning pains in the region of the stomach and liver, sometimes with oppression and vomiting ; diarrhea prostrating, and often involuntarily ; oppression in the chest, with anxious respiration ; delirium, low muttering or talkative ; loss of consciousness.

Dose.—Twelve globules in six tea-spoons of water, a tea-spoonful every hour, or even half-hour, as the symptoms may indicate.

Veratrum.—This remedy is principally indicated in the second and third stage, when there is a general coldness; cramps in the upper and lower extremities, and in the stomach, and abdomen; frequent loose evacuations; dizziness; great thirst; severe vomiting, sometimes of bile and mucus, sometimes of black bile and blood.

Dose.—Twelve globules in six tea-spoonfuls of water, a tea-spoonful every half-hour, hour, or two hours, according to the symptoms.

Diet and Regimen.—Much can be done towards preventing this disease, by paying particular attention to diet and general rules of health. During its prevalence, the food should be plain and simple, highly stimulating articles of diet should be avoided.

Persons should not expose themselves without absolute necessity, in the heat of the day. Change of temperature should be met by change of clothes, and on no condition should persons sleep in damp or confined atmosphere. Diet during convalescence should be the same as in other fevers, as the yellow fever is only a severe form of the bilious fever.

CHAPTER IV.

CUTANEOUS DISEASES.

THE skin is liable to a large number of diseases, more or less severe, some of which affect the whole system, and are accompanied with fever and pain.

Scarlet Fever, Measles, Chicken-Pox, and Small-Pox, are infectious, and generally prevail as epidemics. Very seldom is a person attacked with either of the above diseases more than once.

NETTLE RASH.

The appearance of this rash resembles very much the sting of a nettle. It consists of an irregular pale-red, or whitish eminence, surrounded by a rosy hue. The blotches constantly change their locality, disappearing in a few hours in one part, and appearing in another. Their appearance is preceded by restlessness, and accompanied by burning, itching, and irritation. They are often brought out by cold.

They are occasionied by changes of temperature, imprudence in diet, and in many persons from the use of shell-fish, and some kinds of fruit.

Treatment.—*Dulcamara* may be given if the rash is occasioned by cold, and if preceded by a stinging sensation. Give three globules every six hour.

Aconite.—Will be required when considerable fever is present, and *Rhus*, when it occurs in cold or damp weather, the eruption is of a shining appearance, and attended with some fever. Three globules may be given every three hours.

Bryonia.—May be required when the rash is attended with shivering, or strikes in. Given the same as Rhus.

Ipecac.—Is useful when the rash is accompanied with nausea. Give three globules once in three hours.

Pulsatilla and *Nux-Vomica* are the prominent remedies when the disease is occasioned by indigestion; the former being particularly indicated when the trouble is occasioned by the use of fatty food. Give three globules every six hours.

Calcarea, *Sulphur*, or *Mercurius.*—May be required when the trouble assumes a chronic character. Three globules of the remedy chosen may be given morning and night, changing to another remedy, if, after six doses, no relief is produced.

Diet and Regimen.—Warm bathing, simple food, and no acids.

SCARLET FEVER.

This disease is more generally confined to childhood. The eruption is a bright scarlet rod, turning white on pressure of the finger, resuming its original color on the finger being removed. The eruption is smooth and glossy, unless when combined, as is very often the case, with scarlet rash, when the roughness of the eruption is distinctly felt on passing the hand over the surface. The eruption commences on the face, neck or hands, and gradually spreads over the entire body. The appearance of the eruption is attended with fever, dryness of the mouth, and more or less soreness, or even ulceration, of the throat. As the fever abates, which is usually the case on the fourth or seventh day of the eruption, the eruption gradually disappears and the epidermis peels off in large patches. This disease may be distinguished from measles by the presence of sore throat and the absence of those catarrhal symptoms which are present at the outset of measles.

Treatment.—*Belladonna* is the most important remedy in the treatment of this disease. Its indications are, fever and dryness of the mouth, thirst and sore throat, difficulty of swallowing liquids, shooting in the head, painful eyes, starts, and great nervous excitement.

Dose.—Twelve globules in six tea-spoonfuls of water, a tea-spoonful every two or three hours. If violent fever be present, *Aconite*, prepared in the same manner, should be alternated with the *Belladonna*, one or two hours apart.

Mercurius.—Swelling and ulceration of the throat, with offensive smell and ulceration of the mouth, violent inflammation of the throat.

Dose.—Three globules every two or three hours, alternating with Belladonna, if that remedy is indicated.

After the severity of scarlet fever has subsided, other troubles are likely to be developed. *Pulsatilla* will relieve the violent pain in the ears. Give every two hours.

The running at the ear will be controlled by *Hepar* or *Calcarea*, given three times a day. *Hepar* will also control the hoarse cough, which sometimes follows this disease. Give every three hours.

Diet and Regimen.—As in fever.

MEASLES.

At first the symptoms of an ordinary cold are perceived, such as sneezing, running at the nose, watering of the eyes, short and dry cough, pain in the forehead and back, with more or less fever until the eruption appears.

The eruption appears in the form of small red spots on the face and arms, and gradually extends over the body. On the fourth day the fever begins to abate, and on the sixth or seventh day the skin begins to scale. During the progress of the disease, other troubles may be developed, such as inflammation of the lungs, requiring prompt treatment. Chronic difficulties, often of a tormenting and serious character, not unfrequently follow this disease.

Treatment.—*Aconite and Pulsatilla* are the prominent remedies, and with these the treatment should commence, giving in alternation two or three hours apart.

Dose.—Twelve globules in six tea-spoonfuls of water, a tea-spoonful at a dose.

Bryonia.—May be given when the cough is dry, and there are shooting pain in the chest, difficulty of breathing, and rheumatic pains in the limbs. If fever is present Bryonia may be alternated with Aconite one or two hours apart.

Belladonna.—May be given when there is pain in the head, dry cough, sore throat, twitching of the limbs and restlessness.

Give three globules every two hours.

In the affections which are liable to follow measles, see those particular diseases.

In the severe form of measles and scarlet fever, the room should not be very light, as the eyes are apt to suffer.

Diet and Regimen.—As in fever.

ERYSIPELAS.

Previous to the attack there is usually a general sensation of languor or dullness. In severe cases the parts become very much swollen, the skin presenting a deep red, shining appearance, and the patient suffering severely from a burning heat, tingling, and sensation of tension. The redness and swelling sometimes extend rapidly, and when it appears in the face, as it often does, sometimes covers the entire head.

Sometimes the inflamed surface becomes covered with

little blisters. These severe cases are attended with considerable danger, particularly when the disease attacks the head. There is fever, severe headache, restlessness and sensitiveness to the slightest noise.

Causes.—It may be occasioned by gastric derangement, or by sudden suppression of perspiration, and not unfrequently sets in after mechanical injury.

Treatment.—*Aconite* is indicated when considerable fever is present, with dry and hot skin.

Belladonna.—May be given when the redness expands in rays, and severe shooting pain with great heat is felt, increased by movement; swelling of the face accompanied with burning heat, violent headache, delirium, thirst, and hot skin.

Rhus.—Is particularly indicated when little blisters are perceived, or when there is great swelling, a tendency to spread, or extend to the brain, and when there is great restlessness and delirium.

Dose.—*Belladonna* or *Rhus* may be indicated in alternation with *Aconite.* Twelve globules should be mixed with a glass half full of water, and a teaspoonful given in alternation one or two hours apart. If either of the above remedies are given alone, a dose may be given once in two or three hours.

Pulsatilla.—When the disease affects the ear, when the skin is bluish red, and the spots wander from one place to another, also when the trouble arises from food. Give three globules every three hours.

Diet and Regimen.—Similar to that in fevers. Great

pains should be taken to prevent cold during convalescence.

SMALL POX.

This loathsome disease has ever been looked upon with dread. In England at one time the deaths amounted to 45,000 annually. At length, in 1798, the discovery was made by *Dr. Jenner*, an English physician, that Cow-Pox is almost a sure preservative to Small Pox. Vaccination for Cow-Pox, notwithstanding the ridicule and denunciation with which it was at first received, is now universally adopted, and is the means yearly of saving thousands of lives.

It is well to be revaccinated once in about seven years, to be entirely safe.

Symptoms.—This disease has distinct stages, each of which requires different remedies.

1. *The febrile stage* generally commences from eight to fourteen days after exposure, and continues from two to four days.

It sets in with shivering, fever, and dryness of the skin, hard and frequent pulse, severe pain in the back, and sometimes in the stomach, aching in the bones, and bruised sensation of the flesh, swimming, and severe pain in the head, and sometimes delirium and convulsions. Cough and sensitiveness of the eyes to light, are usually present. Vomiting, and pain in the small of the back are characteristic symptoms of Small-Pox.

2. On the third or fourth day the eruption makes its

appearance on the face, in the form of small, red points, increasing in extent and elevation, and gradually covering the whole body. The eruption is distinguished from others by a small pimple, about the size of a millet-seed, in each point.

3. In the *suppurative stage*, the pustule completes its development, becomes about as large as a split-pea, and is filled with a yellowish fluid, which gradually changes its color, until it assumes a turbid appearance. It is surrounded by a red circle, and has on the top a blackish depression, or dent. The eruption becomes fully developed on one part of the body, while it is only making its appearance on the other. During this stage, which lasts three or four days, more or less fever, swelling, and salivation are present.

4. In the fourth stage the pustules present a brown appearance, and sometimes burst, forming scabs. The fever and swelling gradually subside, the scales peel off, leaving at first a deep, red stain. The *confluent* form of the disease, where the pustules are so numerous as to run into each other, forming an immense scab, is longer in duration, and attended with considerable danger.

Treatment.—The prevention of this fearful disease by vaccination, is purely homeopathic, and its most successful treatment, by which it is deprived of half its dangers, is also homeopathic. The room should be freely ventilated, the patient placed upon a mattress or straw-bed, covered with linen-sheets, and kept cool, and as comfortable as possible.

In the first, or febrile stage, *Aconite* or *Stibium* should, if there is severe pain in the head, intolerance of light, and delirium, be given every two hours.

Belladonna.—May be given in alternation with either of the above remedies, one hour apart.

Bryonia.—Is a valuable remedy, when there is derangement of the stomach, rheumatic pains in the limbs, worse by motion, constipation, shooting pains in the chest on breathing.

Dose.—Twelve globules in six tea-spoons of water, a tea-spoonful every three hours.

Rhus.—Is of benefit when there are rheumatic pains in the back and extremities, worse at night, and relieved by motion ; also great restlessness at night. Give same as *Bryonia.*

Stibium.—Should be given when the cough indicates trouble about the lungs, three globules every two hours.

Stramonium.—In the eruption stage this remedy is of great value in shortening its duration, and is particularly useful when the eruption is slow in its appearance and progress.

Dose.—Twelve globules may be dissolved in a glass half-full of water, and a tea-spoonful given every three hours.

Mercurius.—May be given should there be much salivation. In the last stage simple ablution with tepid water will usually be all that is required.

Diet and Regimen.—The diet should be cooling ; cold water, lemonade, oranges, roasted apples, stewed prunes, strawberries, gruel, and toast, may be used, avoiding the fruits, if diarrhea is present.

VARIOLOID.

This is merely a modified form of Small-Pox, occurring sometimes after vaccination. The treatment is similar to Small Pox.

GENERAL CUTANEOUS DISEASES.

ITCH OR SCABIES.

This very annoying trouble appears in the form of small vesicles, filled with a clear fluid, and surrounded by a red border, between the fingers, on the wrists and in the bend of the joints. Sometimes the eruption extends over the entire body, with the exception of the face. The itching is aggravated in the evening, and by the warmth of the bed. As the vesicles become broken up by scratching they may form thick scabs.

Treatment.—*Sulphur* is the most prominent remedy, and should be taken six globules morning and night for a week.

Mercurius.—May follow the Sulphur, three globules morning and night for a week.

When large boils make their appearance during the progress of the disease, *Silicea* may be given morning and night.

Hepar.—Will be required in those neglected cases, where ulcers have formed. Given three times a day.

Diet and Regimen.—Nourishing food should be freely used, and great cleanliness practiced.

RINGWORM.

This is an eruption which presents the appearance of a ring. Inside, the skin, at first, looks healthy, but gradually becomes rough and scales off as the eruption dies away. It generally occurs in summer, and sometimes disappears in a week, or may last all summer.

Sulphur.—May be given, three globules night and morning for a week. If there is no change for the better, *Graphites* or *Hepar* may be given in the same manner.

TETTER.

There are several varieties of this non-contagious affection of the skin. The eruption consists of vesicles or inflamed patches, and is attended with more or less itching.

Treatment.—Should there be much restlessness and fever, *Rhus* may be given, three globules, morning, noon, and night.

Should the disease assume a dry or scaly character, *Sulphur* or *Silicea* may be given in the same manner, continuing one for three days, when, if no better, proceed with the next remedy.

Mercurius.—May be given as above, when there is a tendency to ulceration.

CHILBLAINS.

This affection is usually confined to the hands and feet, and is the result of cold. They are attended with burning and intense itching. They sometimes ulcerate, when they become exceedingly painful.

Arsenicum.—May be given, three globules every four hours, when there are acute burning pains, and ill-conditioned ulcers.

Nux-Vomica.—May be given in the same manner, if the inflammation is superficial, and attended with slight red swelling.

Pulsatilla.—Will be required should the parts present a blue red and swollen appearance, accompanied with severe throbbing pain. Give three globules, morning, noon and night.

External Applications are often attended with marked benefit. Cloths applied, wrung out in cold water, in the mild form of the complaint, will be of great service. Where this is inconvenient, the afflicted part may be covered with cotton.

Tincture of Arnica.—May be used as a lotion with decided benefit. Twelve drops may be mixed with three table-spoonfuls of water, and the parts bathed three or four times a day; or the feet may be bathed with brandy into which has been dropped a few drops of melted tallow.

WHITLOW—FELON.

An abscess more or less deeply seated, forming about the end of the finger, is called a Felon. The pain, when the disease is fairly developed, is agonizing. The disease may frequently be removed, when it is first noticed, by holding the finger in warm water.

Mercurius.—May be given in the incipient stage, three globules every four hours. But if, after five or six doses, the disease should still advance, *Silicea* and *Hepar* may be give in alternation, four hours apart.

During the progress of the disease, the finger may be either wrapped up in cloths wrung out in cold water, or warm poultices of bread and milk, slippery elm or flax seed, may be applied.

Sometimes, when the disease is attended with intense pain and advances slowly, a free incision may be made with the knife.

ULCERS.

Ulcers may follow a bruise or scald, or when there is a general derangement of the system, occasioned by improper food, they may be openings of nature to carry off the impurities of the system, which might otherwise produce serious disturbance.

Treatment.—Dry soft linen lint may be placed over the ulcer, or it may be covered with a compress, dipped in either cold or warm water, as is most agreeable to the patient.

Arsenicum and *Carbo-v.*—May be given in alternation, three globules of one in the morning and the other in the evening should the ulcer present a livid aspect, bleed readily to the touch, and especially if there is a burning pain.

Mercurius.—May be given, three globules morning and night, if the ulcer is deep, and emits an offensive smell.

Sulphur.—In ulcers of long standing, three globules may be given morning and night.

Cleanliness should be observed, and every pains taken, by means of nourishing food, to build up the general system. The application of the battery, in these cases, may be of benefit. (*See* Electricity.)

BOILS—CARBUNCLES.

A boil is of a round or conical form, having an inflamed appearance, is attended with more or less pain, and suppurates slowly. On breaking, they discharge pus mixed with blood, and after a little while, a core.

There is sometimes a constitutional tendency to boils, but they also often follow fevers and eruptive diseases, and may be occasioned by imprudence in food, either in eating too much or not enough.

Arnica.—Should be given, in most cases, and will often prevent the full development of the boil.

Dose.—Two drops may be mixed with a glass half-full of water, and a tea-spoonful given three times a day.

Hepar or *Mercurius.*—May be given as above, when the matter is forming, to bring it more quickly to a head.

When the boil is painful a poultice should be applied.

The Carbuncle.—Is a malignant kind of boil, and when it occurs on the back of the neck, as is very apt to be the case, is attended with more or less danger. The disease is attended with severe pain and more or less fever. On breaking, the matter is discharged from several openings.

Arsenicum.—Is indicated where there is great prostration of strength. Three globules three times a day.

Hepar and *Silicea.*—Are, however, the prominent remedies, alternated four hours apart. Three globules may be given at a dose.

External application of the cold water compress is generally better than poultices. (*See*, also, Electricity).

ABCESS—SWELLING OF THE GLANDS.

The glands, in different parts of the body, as in the arm-pits, the groins or throat, are liable, from various causes, to swell and suppurate. If there is much heat or pain, the cold water compress, or a poultice may be applied. Three globules of *Mercurius* may also be given once in six hours. This treatment will generally prevent suppuration. Should, however, the swelling still continue, and be slow in its progress, *Hepar* or *Silicea* may be alternated, three globules of one in the morning, and of the other at night.

CHAPTER V.

AFFECTIONS OF THE BRAIN AND NERVOUS SYSTEM.

HEADACHE.

THE head being the seat of the brain, sympathizes with almost every part of the system. To treat headache successfully it is absolutely essential that we should ascertain the cause. Among the numerous varieties of headache we may enumerate, 1. *Nervous Headache.* 2. *Sick Headache.* 3. *Rheumatic Headache.* 4. *Congestive Headache.*

Nervous Headache.—By this we understand that variety when the pain is at first unaccompanied by any disturbance of the stomach. After a time, vomiting may set in, but the substances vomited are generally destitute of bile or acid. This variety of headache includes periodical, neuralgic, one-sided, and certain forms of sick headache. It occurs mostly in persons of a nervous temperament, and is apt to be brought on by any unusual excitement. The pains are of a neuralgic character, violent throbbing, darting and stinging, worse at night, with great sensitiveness to light, noise, or touch.

Sick Headache.—In this variety of headache there is sickness at the stomach, swimming in the head, or violent aching pain, not unfrequently coming on in the morning, and continuing until relieved at night by sleep. Previous derangement of the stomach or bowels is evident, and bile or undigested food is thrown up in the paroxysms of vomiting. The headache generally depends on gastric derangement, and in some persons seems periodical, coming on at intervals, more or less frequent.

Rheumatic Headache.—This form of headache usually comes on in paroxysms, during which the pain is most intense. The slightest motion of the head is attended with pain, and there is a peculiar feeling of constriction over the brain. The urine, as well as the perspiration, is acid.

Congestive Headache.—Some of the prominent symptoms are, violent throbbing of the arteries of the head, fullness and heaviness of the head, accompanied with dizziness, particularly on stooping or walking in the sun; heat in the head, also fullness and pain above the eyes, increased by stooping.

Headache is often the result of constipation, cold, gastric troubles, and external causes.

Treatment.—Ascertain the cause, and strive to avoid it in future. If there is too great a fondness for the pleasures of the table, or any other form of dissipation, strive to live more in accordance with nature. If possessed of a highly excitable nervous organization, banish tea and coffee, and stimulants of all kinds. Whatever may be the cause, live plainly, use cold water freely about the head, and avoid violent physical or mental exertion.

When the headache is caused by *chagrin*, chamomilla may be given.

From *anger: Nux-Vomica.*

From *fright: Opium.*

From *constipation: Nux-Vomica* or *Opium.*

From *gastric derangement: Nux-Vomica, Ipecac, Pulsatilla, or Bryonia.*

From the use of *intoxicating liquor: Nux-Vomica* or *Opium.*

From *a blow: Arnica.*

From *sedentary habits: Nux-Vomica* or *Sulphur.*

Aconite.—Violent headache, accompanied by heat and violent throbbing; heaviness and fullness in the head, compressive pain over the root of the nose, aggravated by noise or motion, relieved in the open air; headache so violent as to produce delirium; one sided headache with nausea and vomiting, and burning pain over the left eye; rheumatic and nervous headache.

Dose.—Twelve globules dissolved in six tea-spoonfuls of water, a tea-spoonful given from one to four hours, according to the severity of the symptoms. If the pain is violent, give every fifteen minutes until relieved. It is often best to alternate with *Belladonna.*

Belladonna.—Headache aggravated by motion, noise, or light; paroxysms of stitching pain on one side; scintillation before the eyes and obscuration of sight. Violent aching or throbbing pain, blood-shot eyes, delirium; pains in the afternoon, aggravated by the warmth of the bed; sudden sharp pains.

Dose.—Same as *Aconite.*

Bryonia.—Compressive pains in the head, or sensation on stooping, as if everything would protrude through the forehead ; aching and pressing pain affecting the fore-head, temples, neck, arms and face.

Dose.—In severe cases, three globules may be given every half-hour, increasing the intervals as the pain abates. In chronic cases, give once in six or twelve hours.

Rhus.—Burning pulsative pains, with fullness in the head ; fluctuation of the brain, as from a fluid rolling inside ; weight in the back part of the head ; nervous headache.

Dose.—Three globules every one, two, or four hours.

Pulsatilla.—Especially indicated in headaches brought on from a derangement of the stomach, produced by the use of indigestible, rich or fat food, from indigestion produced by exertion just before or after a meal ; also from bodily fatigue and loss of rest. Pressure and distressing pain in the side of the head, or attended with dizziness and inclination to vomit, relieved by binding something tight around the head, or walking, and aggravated when quiet or sitting ; heaviness of the head, paleness of the face, and dizziness ; rending pains, worse in the evening ; throbbing, precisely after rising in the morning, and on lying down in the evening. This remedy is particularly indicated in persons of an easy or lymphatic temperament.

Dose.—In severe cases, three globules may be given every half-hour, increasing the intervals as the pain abates, to three or four hours. In chronic cases give three times a day.

Nux-Vomica.—Of great value when the difficulty is caused by abuse of ardent spirits, sedentary mode of life, anger or severe mental labor ; also from constipation and indigestion. Heat and redness of the face; dizziness, violent headache, particularly in the forehead over the eyes, increased by stooping and coughing.

Dose—In severe cases, give three globules every hour. In chronic cases, morning and night.

Mercurius.—Fullness in the head, as if it would split, or as if it were compressed with a band ; worse at night, with burning, tearing pains, easy and profuse perspiration. (*See, also, Cold in the Head.*)

Dose.—Three globules every four or six hours.

Arsenicum.—May be given with benefit in periodical headaches ; face bloated, eyes suffused with tears, lids swollen.

Dose.—Three globules, in severe cases, every two hours ; at longer intervals as the symptoms abate.

Opium.—In congestive headaches, and from fright, also, when there is heaviness and fullness of the head, as if it would burst, increased by the slightest mental exertion, and attended with coldness of the extremities ; sensation of stupor.

Dose.—Three globules in severe cases every half hour ; as the symptoms abate given at longer intervals.

China.—Headache in sensitive persons, when the scalp and face are sensitive to the touch ; violent pain as if the head would burst ; pain aggravated by the slightest movement, and relieved by lying down and by quiet. Give same as *Opium.*

Diet and Regimen.—The application of cold water to the head will be attended with relief. Magnetic passet may be made with the hand over the head with benefit. The food should be easy of digestion, and whatever in the manner of living has a tendency to produce the headache, should be carefully avoided.

DIZZINESS.

This affection seldom exists by itself, but is usually symptomatic.

Belladonna.—Dizziness with sparks before the eyes, or with staggering, nausea, trembling, and recurrence of the attack on stooping or rising up.

Cocculus.—When produced by the motion of a carriage, or by moving the head, with nausea and faintness.

Nux-Vomica.—After a meal, in the open air, or in bed, with wavering in the head, and cloudiness of the eyes.

Pulsatilla.—On raising the eyes, in the evening in bed, or on stooping, or after a meal, with nausea and paleness of the face.

Dose.—Three globules of the appropriate remedy in severe cases every half-hour ; in chronic cases morning and night.

SUN STROKE.

This is an affection of the brain produced by intense

heat. It is very common in warm climates. A person exposed to the intense heat of the sun, may be attacked with dizziness and symptoms closely resembling intoxication, or he may become, almost from the first, perfectly insensible.

The head may be bathed with cold water or brandy; a little brandy given internally will be of benefit; or *Camphor* may be given two drops every ten minutes, to be followed, after four or five doses have been taken by *Belladonna*, three globules at a dose, either alone or in alternation with *Carbo-v.* every half-hour or hour.

INFLAMMATION OF THE BRAIN.

The attack may come on suddenly with stupor and sensitiveness to light; but it is generally attended with severe pain, heat, and fullness in the head, restless sleep, with starting as if in affright. As the disease advances, the pain may become dull and heavy, increased by the slightest movement, head hot and burning, great sensitiveness to light, stupor, delirium, thirst, dry and hot skin.

Treatment.—External application should be made to the head of cold water, frequently removing the cloths, before they become warm. Ice is still better, either in a cloth, or pounded and put in a bladder.

Aconite and *Belladonna* should commence the treatment. Give in alternation, three globules at a dose, one hour apart.

A physician should be consulted as speedily as possible.

APOPLEXY.

Preceding the attack there is generally dullness and heaviness of the head, disposition to sleep, derangement of the memory, slow and full pulse. Sometimes these symptoms are wanting, and the patient falls down without consciousness, totally or partially paralyzed. The pulse is hard, full and slow, speech difficult, and the face livid. In other cases the attack may set with violent headache and vomiting.

A predisposition to apoplexy is indicated by a stout, short body, large and short neck, dark red countenance. The predisposition is increased by rich living and sedentary habits.

Treatment.—Loosen the dress, and place the patient where there is plenty of air. Elevate the head and trunk.

Belladonna.—Severe pain in the forehead, heaviness and dullness of the head, dizziness, snoring breathing, and dilated pupils.

Nux-Vomica.—In the precursory stage in persons of sedentary habits, and addicted to the use of ardent spirits.

Dose.—When the attack has actually commenced, dissolve twelve globules in six tea-spoons of water, and give a tea-spoon every fifteen minutes.

Belladonna.—Should usually commence the treatment.

NEURALGIA.

In speaking of this extremely painful disease, we shall notice, 1. *Neuralgia of the Face.* 2. *Neuralgia of the Heart.*

1. *Neuralgia of the Face.*

The pain comes on in paroxysms at irregular intervals, increasing in intensity until the patient is almost wild. The pain is of a lacerating, tearing, or beating character, and after having lasted a certain length of time, gradually subsides, coming on again, however, in a short time, with even greater intensity. The pain follows the course of the nerves. If it commences at a point in the eyebrow, over the middle of the eye, it may extend to the eyebrows, forehead, and eyes. If it commences at a point about the middle of the cheek-bone, it may extend over the cheek, and radiate to the teeth, palate, and tongue.

Treatment.—*Belladonna* is a prominent remedy in almost every form of facial neuralgia. It is particularly indicated when the pain is aggravated by movement, noise, or the warmth of the bed. Darting pains, twitching of the muscles, and pain in the ball of the eye.

Dose.—During the severity of the attack three globules every half-hour, increasing the intervals to four hours as the symptoms abate.

Colocynth.—Violent, rending, darting pains, occupying chiefly the left side, and aggravated by the slightest touch. Give same as *Belladonna.*

Arsenicum.—When the attacks are periodical, the pain is of a burning, pricking character, around the eyes and in the temple; increased by cold, and temporarily relieved by heat.

Dose.—Same as *Belladonna.*

China.—Particularly in periodical attacks, violent pain, increased by the slightest touch of the skin.

Pulsatilla.—Pain, particularly on one side, worse in the evening, and on lying down, relieved in the open air, feeling of coldness and torpor in the affected side.

Dose.—During the severity of the attack three globules every half-hour. As the symptoms become less violent give once in three or four hours.

2. *Neuralgia of the Heart.*

Violent pain in the region of the heart, coming on in paroxysms, and extending over the chest, arms, and neck.

Treatment.—*Phosphorus.*—When there is intense pain, coldness of the extremities, and great difficulty of breathing.

Arsenicum.—Unable to breath, except with the chest bent forward; oppressive stitching in the region of the heart, renewed by the slightest motion.

Belladonna.—Hurried respiration; shooting, pressing pain in the region of the heart; tremor of the heart, with anguish.

Rhus and *Nux-Vomica.*—May also be indicated.

Dose.—Three globules, if the attack is severe, every ten minutes. Afterwards three times a day.

PARALYSIS.

This affection is very apt to follow Apoplexy. One portion of the body may be completely paralyzed while the other is active. The whole of one side, from the head to the feet, may be paralyzed.

Nux-Vomica.—Especially when the lower extremities are affected ; trembling of the limbs, or heaviness, stiffness, and sensitiveness to cold air ; cramps, and spasmodic twitching of the parts.

Rhus.—Great sensitiveness to cold air, stiffness of the joints. Particularly indicated when caused by nervous fevers. (*See, also, Electricity.*).

Dose.—Three globules three time a day.

DELIRIUM TREMENS.

Unfortunately this disease is so common, that it is very easily recognized. As a general thing it is produced by the long continued use of ardent spirits, although it is sometimes the result of other forms of mental excitement. There is irritability of temper, great restlessness, and usually entire sleeplessness. Talkative delirium, strange, wild fancies, and trembling of the hands.

Treatment.—*Nux-Vomica.*—Trembling of the limbs, twitching of the muscles, delirium. Given at the commencement of the disease, it will often arrest its further progress.

Dose.—Three globules may be given every two or three hours.

Belladonna.—When there is boisterous delirium, congestion of blood to the head, trembling of the limbs.

Opium.—Constant motions; wild and staring expression; tremor of the limbs; frightful visions.

Dose.—Same as *Nux-Vomica.*

Often, when there is hiccough, or great nervous excitement, a cup of coffee will quiet the system.

CHAPTER VI.

AFFECTIONS OF THE EYES AND EARS.

THE eye consists of a globe held in its position by six muscles, attached externally to the *Sclerotic coat*, near the *Cornea*, and internally to the bones of the orbit behind the eye. These muscles produce the various movements of the eyes.

The *sclerotic coat* seen in the white of the eye, is dense and fibrous. It is the strong membrane which invests the ball, except the transparent part in front, which is called the *Cornea*.

Inside of this coat, is the *choroid* coat, which gives the dark color to the pupil. Another coat within the *choroid* is called the *Retina*. The optic nerve passes from the brain through the other coats, and expands on this. This is the seat of vision, where every object we witness, is pictured, and the impression thus transmitted to the brain.

A curtain capable of contraction and dilation, divides the anterior portion of the eye into two chambers. This curtain is called the *Iris*, and the opening in the centre the *Pupil*. The two chambers are filled with a watery humor. Behind this chamber is the *crystalline lens*, and behind the lens a chamber forming a large portion of the ball of the eye, filled with the *Vitreous* humor. Over the eye are the eye-lids, lined on the inside by a delicate membrane, which is also reflected over the ball of the eye, called the *Conjunctiva*. This membrane secretes a fluid which lubricates the eye, and when inflamed presents a blood-shot appearance. At the upper and outer angle of the orbit is the *Lachrymal gland*. It secretes the tears, which, after having passed over the ball of the eye, pass off through small openings at the internal angle, into the nose.

We have then, the *cornea*, collecting and bending inward the rays of light ; the *aqueous* humor transmitting the rays and giving free motion to the *iris;* the *iris* contracting and dilating, admitting only the necessary rays ; the *crystalline lens*, the focus, concentrating the rays, which then, crossing each other, are transmitted through the *vitreous* humor to the *retina*, which serves as a daguerreotype-plate, upon which the image is pictured, and the impression through the expanded optic nerve transmitted to the brain.

INFLAMMATION OF THE EYES.—*Ophthalmia.*

External applications may be made to the eye of cold or tepid water, or of milk and water. If the inflammation is severe, the room should be partially darkened, and the patient kept as quiet as possible. If matter should be secreted, be careful that the towel used for that eye, does not come in contact with the other, or with the eyes of any one else.

When the inflammation is the result of *cold*, it may be attended with more or less cough and fever. The redness gradually extends over the whole eye. The eye is sensitive to the light; burning, shooting pains, and sensation as if sand were lodged between the lids.

Aconite.—Is an important remedy in the commencement, either alone, or in alternation with *Belladonna.*

Belladonna.—Is particularly indicated when there is congestion of the head, redness of the eyes, and sensitiveness to the light.

Dose.—Give three globules every two hours.

In the first stage four drops of *Arnica* may be placed in a glass a third full of water, with which the eye may be bathed.

Rheumatic and Gouty Ophthalmia.—This variety of inflammation is usually connected with rheumatic or gouty troubles in other parts of the system. The pain is intense, sticking, tearing, and boring, frequently extending to the temples, and aggravated by a change of weather. The same treatment is indicated as in catarrhal ophthalmia. *Bryonia*, *Pulsatilla* and *Rhus*, may also be required. (*See Rheumatism.*)

Pulsatilla.—Will be of benefit when, after the first inflammation has been removed by *Aconite*, severe pains of a piercing, cutting character still remain; pains worse in the afternoon and evening.

Dose.—Three globules every two hours.

Colocynth.—Pain, seated in the ball of a burning, cutting character ; pressing, tearing pain in the whole brain, most violent in the forehead on moving the eyes.

Scrofulous sore eyes.—The eye-balls are red and bundles of enlarged vessels run towards the cornea. There is great intolerance of light, increased secretion of mucus, and an aggravation of symptoms towards morning. The lids are also more or less diseased.

Arsenicum.—May be given three globules three times a day, if the pain is of a burning character.

Belladonna.—Sensation of pressure, worse when the eyes are turned upwards. Give three globules three times a day.

Hepar.—Lids sore, and painful to the touch, as if bruised ; spots on the ball, and sensation as if the eyes were pressing from the sockets.

Mercurius.—Eyes congestive and painful ; pustules on the ball ; sensitive to light, and worse in the evening. Give three times a day.

Sulphur.—Is indicated after *Mercurius* or *Hepar*, when the redness and pain still continue ; dimness of the cornea, and a mist before the eyes.

Syphilitic sore eyes.—This variety of inflammation may arise from suppressed gonorrhea or syphilis, and from a transmission of the matter to the eye.

The treatment should commence with *Aconite*, followed after inflammation has somewhat subsided, by *Mercurius*, four globules every four hours.

Other remedies may be indicated, as *Sulphur* or *Nitric*

Acid, but the patient had better at once consult a physician.

Diet and Regimen.—During the severity of the inflammation all stimulating food should be avoided, and the patient should live as directed in fevers.

INFLAMMATION OF THE EYE-LIDS.

The lids are generally more or less affected in inflammation of the eye, but they are sometimes red and swollen when there is no trouble about the eye.

Aconite.—May be given when the swelling is hard, red, with burning heat, and dryness. Give three globules every three hours.

Belladonna.—If the lids stick together, and are red and swollen. Give same as *Aconite.*

Hepar.—A disposition to ulcerate ; pressing pain and soreness. Give morning and night.

Nux-Vomica.—When the edges of the lids burn, itch, and feel sore when touched. Give three globules every four hours.

Mercurius.—When the lids turn outward, and there is pricking, burning, and itching, or an absence of pain. Give same as *Nux-Vomica.*

STYE.

This is a swelling on the edge of the lid like a dark, red boil. It is attended with considerable pain, suppurates, and in a short time breaks.

Pulsatilla.—During the forming stage this remedy will usually be sufficient. Give three globules three times a day.

Should, however, ulceration take place, *Mercurius* or *Hepar* may be given in the same way.

A cold bread and milk poultice, applied over the eye at night, will generally remove the inflammation.

WATERY EYES.

The eyes are suffused with tears, which, instead of passing into the nose by the little ducts opening from the inner end of the lid, flow over the lid. This is occasioned by a stoppage of the tea-ducts, and is more annoying, from the constant necessity of wiping the eye, than painful.

The prominent remedies are *Calcarea*, *Silicea*, and *Sulphur*. Give three globules of the first every morning, for a week, then follow, if necessary, by the other remedies, in the same manner. Bathe the face freely with cold water.

FOREIGN SUBSTANCES IN THE EYE.

Particles of dust can generally be removed by bathing the eyes in cold water. Turn the head one side, and let a few drops of water pass in at the outer part of the eye, and run towards the nose. If the particle be not removed in this way, raise the lid gently, and with the corner of a handkerchief the offending substance can be removed with but little difficulty. If a hard particle should become imbedded in the eye, it may be removed with the point of a needle.

The irritation of the eye may be removed by bathing it with cold water, or with a mixture composed of two drops of *Arnica*, to a table-spoonful of water.

Particles of iron, which among mechanics are very apt to fly into the eye, may be removed with a magnet.

WEAKNESS OF SIGHT.

In case of weakness of sight a careful physician should be consulted. The difficulty may arise from a variety of causes, which would not be apparent except to the physician. The weakness may come on gradually, with or without pain, and be accompanied with numerous symptoms, such as dark spots, flashes of light, or a sensation as of mist before the eyes. The difficulty may be occasioned by other diseases, or be the result of continued watching, mental anxiety, too frequent sexual indulgence, self-pollution, and constant labor of the eyes. Particular attention should be paid to the general health. Food should be nourishing, and, when possible, exercise should be taken in the open air. As it regards the specific treatment, consult a physician.

AFFECTIONS OF THE EARS.

MUMPS.

This disease is not usually dangerous, unless, in its progress, it is thrown upon some other organ. It consists in an inflammation of the large gland lying under and in front of the ears. It seldom attacks a person but once. On the fifth or seventh day the swelling sometimes leaves the neck, and attacks the breast or testicles, which become red and painful.

Treatment.—The patient should remain in the house, keep a handkerchief about the neck, and not take cold.

Mercurius.—In most cases will be all that is necessary. Give three globules three times a day. If the swelling assumes an inflammatory character, resembling erysipelas, and be attended with pain and fever, or should sharp pain be felt in the brain with stupor and delirium, *Belladonna* should be given, three globules every three hours.

If the disease attacks the testicles or the breasts, *Pulsatilla* or *Mercurius* may be given, three globules every three hours.

Carbo-v.—Would be required if the tumor is hard, Mercurius having proved insufficient, or if it recedes, and the stomach or voice be affected. Give three globules every three hours.

INFLAMMATION OF THE EAR.

The inflammation is usually attended with heat, and redness, and swelling, throbbing, and lacerating pain, aggravated by motion, frequently extending over the whole head, and often affecting the brain.

Treatment.—*Pulsatilla*, in ordinary inflammation of the ear, is almost a specific. Give three globules every two hours.

Belladonna.—Will be required should the pain penetrate to the brain, giving indications of severe internal inflammation. If much fever is present, it may be alternated with *Aconite*, one or two hours apart.

Mercurius.—May be required should there be a yellowish discharge from the ear, or a confused noise in the head, with throbbing pain. Give three globules every four hours.

It will be well should there be indications, from a violent, throbbing pain, of gathering in the head, to apply steam. This may be done by filling a tea-pot with warm water, and allowing the steam to pass out of the spout into the ear.

EAR-ACHE.

There is often more or less pain in the ear, sometimes of a neuralgic character, when no inflammation is present.

Arnica.—Will be of service when there is a return of the pain from every exposure.

Belladonna.—Tearing and shooting pains, extending

into the throat ; roaring and humming in the ear, and great sensibility to noise.

Mercurius.—Shooting pains, extending into the teeth and cheek ; pains worse in the evening ; sensation of coldness in the ear.

Nux-Vomica.—Pains extending into the forehead and temples, particularly when the ear-ache occurs in irritable and angry persons.

Pulsatilla.—Where the pain is exceedingly violent, and extends over the whole side of the head.

Dose.—Of the remedy carefully selected, give three globules every two or three hours, according to the severity of the symptoms.

RUNNING OF THE EARS.

This affection is often found in scrofulous persons. It is frequently the result of cold, or may follow other diseases, such as measles, scarlet-fever, or small-pox.

Belladonna.—May be given where it is attended with headache and swelling.

Mercurius.—When the discharge is bloody or offensive, and attended with pricking pain.

Calcarea, Hepar, and *Sulphur,* are indicated where the discharge is tedious.

Dose.—In recent cases three globules of the remedy selected, may be given every six hours. In cases of long standing the remedy may be given once a day for a week, when, if no better, another medicine should be selected.

DEAFNESS.

Hardness of hearing is often connected with other diseases, and will disappear when those are relieved.

Calcarea.—Will be of benefit when there is a sensation as if the ears were obstructed, dryness, or purulent discharge, humming, tinkling, or singing in the ears.

Mercurius.—Rheumatic pain in the ear, tendency to perspiration, sense of obstruction, ceasing when swallowing, or blowing the nose.

Pulsatilla.—Tinkling or chirping, sensation of stoppage, roaring, or humming.

Sulphur.—Obstruction of the ears, particularly upon swallowing, gurgling as if caused by water, or humming, and roaring.

Carbo-v.—Chirping, humming, or musical sound in the ear.

Dose.—Give three globules morning and night.

If there is a dryness of the ear, occasioned by hardened ear-wax, let it be carefully removed.

CHAPTER VII.

AFFECTIONS OF THE MOUTH AND THROAT.

TOOTH-ACHE.

To insure healthy teeth they should be brushed in the morning, after each meal, and at night, and the mouth kept sweet and clean by rinsing it with cold water. Avoid also exposing them to sudden changes of heat and cold, as drinking cold water when the mouth is filled with hot food.

Decayed teeth are often occasioned by an unhealthy state of the stomach, and also under allopathic treatment, by taking large quantities of acid and minerals. If the teeth become diseased, consult a skillful dentist, and do not be too anxious to have them extracted, because of a little pain. They may often be preserved by filling, if not ulcerated at the roots, even if very much decayed.

Treatment.—*Aconite* may be given if considerable fever is present.

Belladonna.—Severe pain in the teeth, face, and ears, worse at night; swelling of the gums and cheek, pains worse in the open air, from contact or mental exertion.

Chamomilla.—Violent pain, worse at night, from the warmth of the bed, redness and swelling of the face; pain sometimes affecting the whole side of the face, increased by eating or drinking.

Mercurius.—Severe pain in the roots of the teeth, increased by the warmth of the bed, or by damp air, and by eating and drinking; sometimes affecting the entire side of the face, extending into the ear and glands; sensation as if the teeth were too long; ulceration and bleeding of the gums.

Pulsatilla.—In persons of a mild and timid disposition, especially when the pain is on one side, or is accompanied with ear-ache and headache. Relieved by chewing, by cold water, or cold air.

Nux-Vomica.—In persons accustomed to the use of coffee, ardent spirits, or who live a sedentary life, swelling of the glands, chillness, and sometimes pain in the head, back, and limbs.

Dose.—Give three globules, where the pain is severe, every hour, increasing the intervals as the symptoms abate.

OFFENSIVE BREATH.

This usually arises from decayed teeth, or a deranged state of the stomach. (See *Toothache* and *Dyspepsia.*)

SCURVY.

This affection is more common among sailors, who have been for a long time without fresh provisions, and also among those who have been accustomed to scanty and unhealthy food.

There is fetor of the breath ; the gums are spongy, and inclined to bleed, or ulcerate. They often recede, so that the teeth may be picked out with the fingers. As the disease advances it affects the whole body, producing ulceration and swelling of the limbs.

Treatment.—A healthy, nourishing diet will often produce a cure. Fruits, vegetables, lemon-juice, and other acid drinks, should be used. Potatoes are also exceedingly beneficial as an article of diet.

Mercurius.—Where the gums are red and spongy, ulcerated, and bleeding, with burning pains at night. Fetid smell from the mouth, ulceration of the tongue.

Carbo-v.—May be given where Mercurius does not seem to produce relief, and there are pains, bleeding, and ulceration of the gums, looseness of the teeth, and ulcers in the mouth.

Arsenicum.—Severe ulceration with violent burning pain and prostration.

Dose.—Three globules may be given four times a day.

Diet and Regimen.—Until the severity of the disease has subsided, the diet should be of a farinaceous or vegetable form. The mouth may be rinsed with lemonade, brandy and water, or a little borax and water.

SORE THROAT—QUINSY.

Sore throat may be attended with but little pain, and

slight inflammation, or the swelling may be so great as almost to choke up the passage, and be attended with fever, pain, and, if not relieved, ulceration.

Treatment.—In the commencement of this disease a cloth wrung out in cold water, placed around the throat, and over this a dry flannel, will be of great service. Persons predisposed to throat-difficulties, should allow the hair to grow around the throat, and sponge the throat and upper portion of the chest with cold water.

The treatment can usually commence with *Belladonna*, three globules given every two or three hours.

Aconite.—Violent fever, thirst, difficulty of swallowing. Alternate it with Belladonna or Mercurius.

Belladonna.—One of the most prominent remedies in all forms of sore throat; swelling on the outside of the throat, constant disposition to swallow, producing severe pain; spasms of the throat when drinking, fluids passing through the nose; sensation as of a plug in the throat; swelling and redness of the parts, and shooting pains in the throat.

Dose.—Give three globules every two hours.

Mercurius.—Redness and swelling of the throat, shooting pains in the throat, especially on swallowing, extending to the ears and glands of the neck; painful and difficult swallowing, ulcers, and tendency to suppuration; profuse discharge of saliva, symptoms worse at night, or in the open air.

Dose.—Three globules every two hours, or alternate with Belladonna, one, two, or three hours apart, according to the severity of the symptoms.

Nux-Vomica.—Sensation of a lump in the throat when swallowing, and pressing pains aggravated by swallowing; throat feels raw and excoriated, as if scraped.

Dose.—Give three globules every three hours.

Pulsatilla.—Persons of a timid or mild character; redness of the throat, a sensation as if the parts were swollen ; scraping pain, and dryness in the throat, without thirst.

Dose.—Three globules every two hours.

Bryonia.—Dry cough, and oppressed respiration, painful sensibility of the throat when touched, on turning the head, or swallowing.

Dose.—Give the same as Pulsatilla.

Cantharides.—Burning and grating, or smarting of the throat ; difficulty in swallowing liquids, tickling in the throat ; dry cough, followed by distressing respiration, and sometimes bloody expectoration.

Dose.—Three globules every two hours.

Hepar.—Where the tonsils are very much swollen this remedy will often accelerate suppuration.

Dose.—Give three globules every three hours.

In *malignant* or *putrid sore throat* the disease may set in with great violence, and run its course in a short time.

Arsenicum.—Is particularly indicated where there is great prostration of strength, fetid smell from the mouth, great restlessness, and anguish. Give three globules every three hours.

(See the preceding remedies. Consult also *Scarletina.*)

CHAPTER VIII.

AFFECTIONS OF THE STOMACH AND BOWELS.

DYSPEPSIA.

OWING to our artificial manner of living, this is by no means an uncommon disease. Did we live in perfect obedience to nature's laws, partaking of food at proper times, and in kind and quantity only what the system requires, we should escape a host of troublesome ailments, which fill our system with pain, and not unfrequently shorten our days.

The stomach, crowded with rich food taken at all hours, or deprived of what is essential to the nourishment of the body, of a necessity becomes weak and inactive, and utters its warnings in pain more or less severe, fretfulness of disposition, and a general derangement of the entire system, as almost every organ in the body sympathizes with the stomach.

Dyspepsia may be produced by taking too much and too rich food, by not enough, by eating at irregular hours, or eating too great a variety at one time ; by indulging in the free use of stimulants, tobacco, coffee, and from various other causes.

Symptoms.—A sensation of weight in the stomach, or

a fullness and heaviness, especially after eating, appetite capricious, flatulence, belching of wind, nausea, and sometimes vomiting of acid or bitter fluids ; drowsiness, particularly after eating ; depression of spirits, and a general sense of uneasiness.

Treatment.—Stimulants, such as ardent spirits, spices or tobacco, only produce a temporary relief, and should therefore be avoided. Food easy of digestion, a little at a time, and taken at regular intervals, will give the stomach time to act, and often gradually enable it to regain its natural strength.

Recent cases of dyspepsia are generally controlled by means of *Pulsatilla*, *Ipecac*, or *Nux-Vomica*.

Nux-Vomica.—Particularly indicated where there is a predisposition to piles, and constipation, in persons of an irritable or lively temperament, and at the commencement of the treatment. Unpleasant taste in the mouth, hunger, or repugnance to food ; nausea, or sour eructations, flatulence, headache, and disposition to sleep, sensation of fullness about the stomach, constipation. This remedy is particularly useful where the sufferings are the result of various forms of dissipation.

Dose.—In severe cases three globules every four hours; in cases of long standing give night and morning.

Sulphur.—Especially in the beginning of the treatment and in chronic dyspepsia. There is a repugnance to food, pain in the stomach after eating, craving for acids, and acidity of the stomach.

Dose.—Give the same as Nux, with which, in chronic

cases, it may be alternated--three globules of the Sulphur being taken in the morning, and three of the Nux at night.

Pulsatilla.—Particularly useful where the disease has been occasioned by fatty food; there is craving for acids and rich food; nausea, eructations, and oftentimes colic and diarrhea.

Dose.—Give three globules every three hours.

Bryonia.—Particularly useful in damp weather, and where there is constipation; painful sensibility of the stomach to the touch, and a sense of fullness; vomiting of food after a meal; craving for stimulants, and aversion to food or morbid appetite.

Dose.—Same as Pulsatilla.

Ipecac.—Tongue furred with white or yellowish coating, insipid, clammy taste, nausea, and vomiting.

Dose.—Give three globules every two hours.

China.—Particularly in marshy districts, and where the system has been weakened by blood-letting and purging; indifference to food, and craving for stimulants, great weakness, drowsiness, and sensibility to currents of air.

Dose.—Give three globules every four hours.

Mercurius.—Unpleasant taste in the morning, constipation with straining; painful sensibility of the stomach.

Dose.—Give three globules morning and night.

Arsenicum.—Stomach sensitive to the touch; fullness or aching sensation; burning pains, or colic in the stomach, sometimes with chillness and anguish; great debi lity, nausea, vomiting, and diarrhea, particularly after drinking.

Dose.—Give three globules every three or four hours.

Diet and Regimen.—Stimulants, and rich or highly-seasoned food, should be avoided; simple food, plainly cooked, should be taken in moderate quantities at regular intervals; drink but little at meals; do not eat heartily when very much fatigued, and do not commence violent labor, either physical or intellectual, within half an hour after eating; use moderate exercise in the open air; cultivate cheerful conversation, and avoid unpleasant or gloomy thoughts; avoid dissipation of all kinds, and conform to the simple teaching of nature. By following these directions Dyspepsia, that fruitful source of a host of pains and torturing diseases, may be often removed with but little, if any medicine. (See, also *Exercise*, page 43; also from page 18 to 25.)

NAUSEA AND VOMITING.

These difficulties are sometimes the result of errors in diet, although, as a general thing, they occur in the progress of other diseases.

(See *Dyspepsia—Fevers.*)

Ipecac.—In simple nausea or vomiting will generally produce relief.

Pulsatilla.—Is particularly useful in females, and in nausea occasioned by the use of fatty food.

Nux-Vomica.—When the vomiting is the result of dissipation.

Cocculus or *Pulsatilla.*—When occasioned by the motion of a carriage, or from being on the water.

Dose.—Three globules may be given every half-hour, hour, or two hours, according to the severity of the symptoms.

SEA-SICKNESS.

A description of sea-sickness would require the pen of a poet to do it justice. The retching and vomiting, the intense nausea, the disregard of life, and the lengthened visage, often furnish food for mirth to those who, from being frequently on the sea, or from other causes, escape entirely or in part, this annoying sickness.

The severity and duration of this sickness depend in a great measure, upon temperament and the condition of the person at the time. Some are sick from the motion of a carriage, or when the water is but slightly disturbed, while others experience no trouble even in the wildest storms of the ocean.

Treatment.—The patient should remain as much as possible in the open air, and for the first few days avoid eating heartily. The confined air of the cabins or state-room is apt to increase the difficulty. Some obtain relief by drawing a bandage tightly around the body, just below the stomach.

Three globules of Nux-Vomica taken on embarking will often prevent an attack.

Cocculus.—With nausea, extreme sensitiveness of smell; loathing of smoking; hunger, but no appetite. This remedy is also particularly servicable for the nausea occasioned by the motion of a carriage.

Dose.—Give three globules, at first every half-hour, until three doses have been taken, afterwards every hour or two hours.

Arsenicum.—May follow *Cocculus*, if the sickness becomes excessive, and is attended with great prostration, violent retching and vomiting, burning sensation in the throat or stomach.

Dose.—Give three globules during the interval between the paroxysm, until relief is obtained, or another remedy is indicated.

Nux-Vomica.—Particularly serviceable in persons of a bilious or nervous temperament, or in alternation with *Cocculus*, after *Arsenicum* has been given with benefit, to dissipate the sensations of swimming and nausea, which may remain. It may also be given in alternation with *Arsenicum*, particularly when the symptoms are slight, and commence soon after embarking.

Dose.—If given alone, give three globules every two hours; if in alternation with *Cocculus*, one hour apart; if in alternation with *Arsenicum*, two hours apart.

Ipecac.—Will be of benefit when the vomiting is free and unattended with prostration of strength. It is also of service when there is no vomiting, but constant and distressing nausea. Give three globules every hour until relieved.

SPASMS AND PAIN IN THE STOMACH.

This affection is characterized by pain, more or less severe, in the region of the stomach. Sometimes the pain is very light, or dull and heavy, at others violently constrictive, cutting, or tearing, making the patient bend double. Hard pressure from without generally relieves the pain. The paroxysms vary in duration, and are often attended by vomiting, flatulence, hiccough, constipation, and palpitation of the heart. This disease may be occasioned by the same causes which produce Dyspepsia, viz., errors of diet, dissipation, &c.

Treatment.—Apply externally hot cloths, or even a warm poultice.

Nux-Vomica.—Is a valuable remedy, especially at the commencement of the disease. There is flatulence, oppression of the chest, contractive, pressive, and spasmodic pain ; nausea, and water-brash ; changeable disposition ; palpitation of the heart.

Dose.—In acute cases three globules every hour ; in chronic cases morning and night.

Carbo-v.—After *Nux*, and when there is violent contractive spasmodic pain, worse on lying down ; flatulence, burning pressure, worse at night, or after a meal.

Dose.—Give same as *Nux.*

Cocculus.—When *Nux* fails to produce relief.

Pulsatilla.—Pain, either from fasting or overloading the stomach, with nausea and vomiting ; shooting pains, increased by walking, and in the evening.

Dose.—Give same as *Nux.*

Bryonia.—In the milder forms of the disease; pressure in the pit of the stomach, with sensation of swelling, headache, constipation. Give three globules every three hours.

China.—Is indicated when the disease is occasioned by debility.

Arsenicum.—When there is prostration, burning pain, vomiting on drinking the smallest quantity.

COLIC.

Colic is characterized by griping, tearing, or cutting pain, more or less severe, coming on in paroxysms in different parts of the abdomen. The pain is often very violent, is relieved by pressure, and is often attended by nausea and vomiting. The absence of fever, except in violent paroxysms, the pain being relieved by pressure, and the quiet, soft pulse distinguish colic from inflammation of the bowels.

Colic may be produced by dissipation, errors in diet, cold, and any of the causes which have a tendency to derange the stomach and abdomen.

Flatulent Colic.—Is often present in persons suffering from dyspepsia, or in those who have been poorly nourished, or who have been accustomed to the free use of spirits.

Bilious Colic.—Preceding this form of colic there are usually symptoms of disordered stomach, such as bitter taste, yellow fur on the tongue, nausea, thirst, restlessness, severe, cutting, writhing pain. In short time vomiting supervenes ; the bowels are freely moved, when the symptoms gradually abate, and as a general thing the patient rapidly recovers.

Painters' Colic.—This disease is occasioned by being exposed to the action of lead, and is very common among painters who use white-lead in their paint, as well as among plumbers, and those engaged in smelting-ores and in lead manufactories. At first, there is loss of appetite, restless nights, and disturbance of the nervous system; this is followed by vomiting, pain in the abdomen, at first in paroxysms, but gradually increasing, until it becomes almost constant. There is little or no fever, but headache, pain in the limbs, obstinate constipation, and after the severe symptoms have passed away, sometimes paralysis of the extremities. An almost invariable symptom of Lead-Colic is a bluish line, extending along the edge of the gums ; sometimes this bluish tinge extends over the mouth.

Treatment.—A warm bath will often produce speedy relief. If convenient the patient may be seated in the bath, the water coming up to the stomach, the upper part of the body being covered so as to confine the steam, and permitted to remain in this situation ten or twelve minutes. He can then be taken out and covered warm in the bed, bottles of hot water being placed to the feet. When this form of bath is not convenient, warm cloths can be placed over the abdomen.

Nux-Vomica—Constipation, pressure in the abdomen

as from a stone, with flatulence, pinching or contractive pains, fullness and tension in the stomach and abdomen, griping and flatulence, pain in the loins, and pressive headache, numbness during pain.

Dose.—Give three globules every half-hour, until relieved, or a change of remedies is indicated.

Colcoynth.—Violent cutting and griping pains, bruised sensation, and tenderness of the abdomen, constipation, or diarrhea, and bilious vomiting after eating.

Dose.—The same as Nux.

Pulsatilla.—Stinging pains in the bowels, and throbbing at the pit of the stomach ; heaviness, fullness, tightness, or bruised sensation in the stomach and abdomen, incarcerated wind, with rumbling and griping, sore and bruised sensation of the bowels when touched ; pains worse in the evening, on lying down, and relieved by walking about; pain in the small of the back when rising, nausea, diarrhea, pressive headache.

Dose.—Give three globules every hour until relieved.

Belladonna.—Violent pain in the stomach and bowels, as if the intestines were grasped by the finger-nails ; or spasmodic constriction in the bowels, with burning and pressure in the small of the back ; redness of the face, and pain in the head.

Dose—Give three globules every half-hour until relieved, or a change of remedy is indicated.

Cocculus.—Colic attended with constipation, with rumbling of flatulence ; spasmodic pains, nausea, shortness of breath, and distention of the stomach ; sensation of emptiness in the abdomen, tearing and burning in the bowels, with clawing in the stomach, nervous excitability.

Dose.—Give the same as *Belladonna.*

China.—Especially useful in flatulent colic, in debilitated persons, and also where the pain appears at night.

Dose.—Give three globules every hour.

Arsenicum.—Violent pain with great anguish, sensation of burning or of cold in the abdomen, nausea, or vomiting.

Dose.—Three globules every two hours.

Mercurius.—Tenderness of the abdomen when touched; pains worse after midnight; nausea, water rising in the throat, or slimy diarrhea ; violent pains, especially around the navel, with distention and hardness of the abdomen, morbid appetite.

Dose.—Give three globules every hour, until three doses have been given, when, if not relieved, follow with *Sulphur* in the same manner.

Diet and Regimen.—The food should be easy of digestion, carefully avoiding all flatulent diet.

In violent cases of flatulent or bilious colic, where the bowels are constipated, it may be necessary to administer an injection. This may consist of about a pint of lukewarm water, administered with an ordinary syringe. In these cases also, the colic is often relieved by drinking freely of warm water sweetened with molasses.

JAUNDICE.

This disease may be either acute or chronic, and continue from a few days to several weeks.

The liver is inactive and does not secrete the necessary amount of bile. Hence the bile, instead of being taken up by the liver, passes through the system, giving a yellow color to the skin. There is a bitter taste, and sometimes nausea, distended abdomen, and pain in the region of the liver. This affection is frequently the result of errors of diet, and from the abuse of quinine and cathartics. It may also follow Intermittent Fever.

Treatment.—The patient should be kept in a warm, and even temperature and perspiration encouraged. Warm bathing, or the application of a bandage wrung out in cold water, around the body in the region of the liver, and this covered with a dry bandage, will often be of service.

Mercurius.—Is a prominent remedy in almost all forms of this disease. Especially when it seems to have arisen from the digestive organs ; pain in the region of the liver.

Dose.—Give three globules three times a day.

China.—Will be of benefit when the disease arises from the abuse of Mercury, and also where there is pressure at the stomach, distention of the abdomen, nausea. diarrhea, and great debility. Give the same as *Mercurius.*

Nux-Vomica.—When occasioned by chagrin and anger, by abuse of spirits, coffee, or tobacco, also by sudden changes of temperature.

Dose.—Give three globules three times a day.

Pulsatilla.—Espesially after abuse of China, and from overloaded stomach, unpleasant dreams, and restlessness at night; bitter taste in the mouth, bilious vomiting, throbbing in the pit of the stomach.

Dose.—Give three globules every four hours.

Either of the above remedies may be given in acute cases every three or four hours, in chronic cases three times a day.

Diet and Regimen.—Farinaceous food, fruits, &c., and in chronic cases meat simply cooked.

DIARRHEA.

Diarrhea consists of loose evacuations from the bowels, more or less frequent, and brought on by various causes. It may be produced by cold, suppressed perspiration, fright, or fear, and by disordered state of the stomach.

Diarrhea is not unfrequently developed during the progress of serious diseases; it sometimes indicates a favorable *crisis*, at others the rapid prostration of the system. When it is a favorable symptom there is a decrease of fever, and a more even, and quiet circulation.

Much harm is often done by means of cathartic, which, acting powerfully on the already weakened intestinal canal, weakens it still more. A free use of astringents and narcotics, such as opium, or sugar of lead, may check the diarrhea, but in so doing the cause is not removed and that, still acting, may develop a more serious affection in some other organ.

The object of the remedy should be to remove irritation, and bring back the weakened intestinal canal to its original strength.

Treatment.—*Dulcamara.*—Is especially indicated when the diarrhea has been occasioned by cold, and the evacuations are of a green, yellow, sour, or slimy character, occurring particularly at night, and often accompanied with cutting pain.

Dose.—Give three globules every three, four, or six hours.

China.—If the diarrhea be of a debilitating kind, occurring particularly at night, or after eating, and containing undigested food.

Dose.—Give morning, noon, and night.

Arsenicum.—Evacuations of a watery, slimy, bilious, putrid, or brownish character, with burning or tearing pains, especially after midnight, thirst, vomiting, and great prostration ; pale face, distention of the abdomen, and coldness of the extremities.

Dose.—In violent cases three globules may be given every hour, until relieved.

Bryonia.—Especially during the heat of summer, or when produced by drinking cold water, by vexation, fright, or a fit of passion.

Dose.—Give three globules every three hours.

Colocynth.—Bilious or watery diarrhea, with spasmodic

colic, and violent, griping pain, particularly when caused by vexation or passion.

Dose.—Give three globules every hour or two hours, until relieved.

Chamomilla.—Slimy, bilious, or watery diarrhoa, yellowish or greenish, resembling chopped eggs ; want of appetite, rumbling in the bowels ; tearing, griping pain, fullness of the stomach, and sometimes bilious vomiting. Give same as *Colocynth.*

Ipecac.—Watery diarrhea, with nausea, vomiting ; bloody or slimy diarrhea, with tearing, colic, and restlessness.

Dose.—Give every two hours.

Pulsatilla.—Particularly when occasioned by a disordered stomach, and the stools are of a watery, greenish, or slimy character, accompanied by cutting pain ; worse at night. Give same as *Ipecac.*

Mercurius.—Evacuations of a watery, bilious, slimy, or frothy character, or greenish and bloody, preceded by colic and griping, and followed by straining, burning, itching, and excoriation of the anus, nausea, and shivering.

Dose.—Give three globules every three hours.

Nux-Vomica.—Frequent but scanty evacuations, with griping pain, colic, and straining. Give as above.

Phosphorus.—In chronic diarrhea, with painless evacuations and emaciation. Give morning and night.

Veratrum.—Diarrhea resembling cholera (which see), or where there are cramp-like or cutting pains and debility.

Diet and Regimen.—In severe cases rest is advisable. The diet should consist of light, unirritating food, such as toast, farina, or arrow-root, except in chronic cases, where it may be more nourishing, yet easy of digestion. Fruits and acid drinks should generally be avoided, except perhaps in bilious diarrheas, occurring during the heat of summer, when a little of some slightly acid drinks, such as cider, or weak lemonade, will often produce not only marked relief, but a complete cure.

DYSENTERY—BLOODY FLUX.

This disease is intensely painful, and requires prompt and vigorous treatment. It is generally attended with fever, and sometimes headache, nausea, and vomiting. Preceding the attack there is usually a loss of appetite, constipation, or diarrhea. These symptoms are soon followed by evacuations of mucus, then mucus mixed with blood, and sometimes pure blood, with almost constant desire for stool, violent straining, and intense pain. The discharge at times is of a whitish or jelly-like mucus, resembling the scraping of the intestines, or green, black, and fetid, or perhaps pure blood. It may be occasioned by indigestible food, decayed or unripe fruits, abuse of spirituous liquors, or sudden suppression of perspiration. It often prevails to an alarming extent in damp, marshy districts, and is most violent in the summer and autumn.

Treatment.—*Aconite.*—Is indicated in the commencement, where there are fever, shivering, heat, and thirst, with rheumatic pains in the head, neck, and shoulders, watery or bilious evacuations, sometimes tinged with blood; dull, or cutting pain in the bowels.

Dose.—Give three globules every two or three hours, until relieved, or another remedy is indicated.

Belladonna.—May be given after, or in alternation with *Aconite*, where in addition to the fever the symptoms are worse in the afternoon, the patient restless, the face red, and the head hot.

Dose.—The same as *Aconite.*

Mercurius.—Is one of the most valuable remedies in the treatment of this disease. Violent straining, with bearing down pain, as if the intestines would be forced out, which only produces a passage of blood, or blood mixed with a substance resembling chopped eggs. During, or preceding the evacutions, there may be nausea, colic, or shivering.

Colocynth.—Bloody stools, fullness and pressure in the bowels, and particularly severe griping colic, sometimes so violent as to cause the patient to bend double.

Dose.—*Colocynth* and *Mercurius* are often indicated at the same time, when they may be given in alternation, three globules one, two, or three hours apart. When either is given alone, three globules may be taken every two or three hours.

Ipecac.—Is particularly useful in Fall Dysentery, where there is nausea, straining, and colic, with stools first of a slimy, then of bloody mucus.

Dose.—Give three globules every two or three hours.

Arsenicum.—Burning pain in evacuating the bowels, rapid prostration of strength, coldness of the extremities, putrid and offensive discharges, which are often involuntary.

Dose.—Give three globules every two or three hours.

China.—Where the disease occurs in marshy countries, and is accompanied with great prostration of strength.

Dose.—Give every three hours.

Nux-Vomica.—Small, frequent evacuations, with straining and cutting pain about the navel; particularly useful when brought on by the heat of summer.

Dose.—Give the same as *China.*

Sulphur.—After other remedies have failed, a few doses of *Sulphur* given at intervals of three or four hours, will often produce relief.

Diet.—All animal food should be avoided; the patient should keep in a reclining posture, in a well-ventilated room; the food and drink should consist of cold water, toast water, rice coffee, arrow-root, farina, and gruel.

CHOLERA MORBUS.

This disease occurs principally in summer and autumn, and runs its course rapidly. It may be preceded by languor and nausea, but it generally comes on suddenly. There is nausea, violent vomiting, and purging, accompanied with cutting and griping colic, particularly about the navel. In the severe form of this disease there may be cramps in the extremities, cold, and clammy skin, and great prostration.

The disease is occasioned by taking cold suddenly in hot weather, exposure to long-continued heat, and food of an unhealthy character.

Ipecac.—May be given in the commencement of this disease, where there is nausea and vomiting.

Veratrum.—Should be given if, notwithstanding *Ipecac*, the disease still advances; the vomiting and diarrhea are violent, the abdomen is tender to the touch; there are violent pains in the region of the navel, and sometimes cramps in the extremities.

Arsenicum.—Is indicated where the disease commences with violence, and is attended with rapid prostration of strength.

Colocynth.—Is also a valuable remedy where there is violet griping colic, and bilious vomiting.

Dose.—Three globules may be given where the symptoms are violent, every twenty minutes, increasing the intervals when the unpleasant symptoms abate.

Diet and Regimen.—Dry, hot clothes should be applied to the abdomen, the patient kept warm by means of blankets, and perhaps bottles of hot water to the feet.

ASIATIC CHOLERA.

This fearful disease sometimes sets in without any perceptible premonitory symptoms, and runs its course in a few hours. There are, however, usually premonitory symptoms, such as general uneasiness, dizziness, rumbling in the bowels, and diarrhea.

As the disease becomes fully developed, there is violent vomiting and diarrhea, and rapid prostration of strength. After a few evacuations the diarrhea presents the appearance of rice-water, and is without smell. There is a painful, burning sensation in the stomach, intense thirst, fearful cramps in the bowels and extremities, and great restlessness. The face presents a sunken appearance, the voice is hollow, and the extremities cold.

The predisposing causes are undoubtedly unripe fruit, indigestible and unwholesome food, dissipation, by which the system loses its vital force, badly ventilated rooms, impure air, occasioned by decaying animal or vegetable matter, and any cause which has a tendency to derange the stomach or bowels, or greatly fatigue or excite the mind or body. When this disease prevails people should live as temperate as possible, avoiding unnecessary fatigue or excitement. Further than this no particular change should be made in living, except that the fruit and vegetables should be ripe and fresh, and the food easy of digestion.

Treatment.—*Camphor* is the great specific in the first stage. The vomiting and rice-water discharges will not unfrequently be entirely checked by a few doses of this remedy. Cover the patient up warm in bed, apply warmth to the feet, and give one drop of the tincture of *Camphor* in a little water every three, five, or ten minutes, until a genial warmth begins to pervade the system, when it may be given less frequently, and when a full perspiration commences cease entirely. A little brandy and water may now be given ; if headache should follow the use of *Camphor*, give three globules of *Belladonna*; should, however, cramps commence in the extremities or bowels, the diarrhea still continuing, *Veratrum* should be given, six globules every ten or fifteen minutes. If there is great oppression and spasmodic constriction about the chest, *Cuprum* will be required, given the same as *Veratrum*, with which it can generally be alternated, ten or fifteen minutes apart.

Should the disease pass into the stage of collapse, indicated by complete prostration, general coldness, and burning sensation in the stomach, and the above remedies have been used, three globules of *Arsenicum* may be given every half-hour.

During the progress of the disease small lumps of ice may be held in the mouth, external warmth in the early stage should be applied in the form of warm blankets, or bottles of hot water, and the limbs should be rubbed with the dry hand.

For the precursory symptoms, such as diarrhea, headache, &c., consult those diseases.

Diet and Regimen.—As the severity of the disease subsides, a little brandy and water may be given, or a little broth, gradually returning to the old diet.

CONSTIPATION.

Constipation often exists in connection with some other

disease. It is usually occasioned by a deranged state of the stomach, or inaction of the liver and bowels. It frequently exists in persons who lead a sedentary life, taking but little exercise, and is also the result of dissipation, and irregularity in eating. It can usually be remedied by exercise, and food of opening character, such as fruit and vegetables. (See *Exercise*, page 43 ; *Food*, page 19.)

Treatment.—Cathartics should be avoided, as they have a tendency, by weakening the bowels, to increase the difficulty. Injections can be used where mechanical means are required.

Nux-Vomica.—Is a valuable remedy, especially in chronic cases, occasioned by dissipation, sedentary habits, or indigestible food. There may be, aside from the constipation, headache.

Dose.—Six globules may be given at night, and six of *Sulphur* in the morning for a week if necessary.

Opium.—Is of benefit in more recent cases, when occasioned by sedentary habits, and where there is fullness about the head.

Dose.—Give three globules morning and night.

In chronic cases the sitz-bath is a valuable help, also bathing the abdomen freely with cold water. After the bowels have become strong, a stated hour every day for going to stool, exercise, and proper attention to diet, will prevent all further difficulty.

PILES.

These are small tumours or lumps just within the rectum; they sometimes bleed, and, at other times, their presence is only indicated by a sense of fullness and pain. They are often occasioned by constipation, also by the free use of cathartics under Allopathic treatment.

The sitz-bath is of great benefit. The patient seating himself in a tub of cold water, the water coming up around the hips, and remaining in that position for three or four minutes.

Nux-Vomica.—Is of benefit when occasioned by constipation, errors of diet, or sedentary life. It may be given six pellets at night, and six of *Sulphur* in the morning.

Belladonna.—May be given in alternation with *Arnica*, two or three hours apart, where there is severe pain in the small of the back, and discharge of blood.

CHAPTER IX.

URINARY AND GENITAL ORGANS.

The kidneys, whose office it is to secrete the urine, are located on either side of the spine, just below the last false rib. The urine is conveyed from each kidney by a small tube to the bladder. The bladder is the reservoir for the urine, and is situated in the lower part of the abdomen.

INFLAMMATION OF THE BLADDER.

In inflammation of the bladder there are chills, fever, and sometimes nausea. The urine is discharged drop by drop, is thick, dark red, and there is more or less pain in the region of the bladder. Should there be much fever, and difficulty in passing water, *Aconite* should be given in alternation with *Cantharides*, every one, two, or three hours.

Nux.—Will be found of benefit when occasioned by abuse of spirituous liquors. Give every three or four hours. Avoid wines and liquors, and all kinds of stimulating food. The same treatment may be pursued in Inflammation of the Kidneys.

SUPPRESSION AND RETENTION OF URINE.

These affections generally exist in connection with some other disease, and should receive prompt attention. In suppression of the urine there is no secretion, while in retention, the urine is secreted, but, owing to a weakened state of the neck of the bladder, or some mechanical cause, it is not discharged. Warm or cold cloths may be applied over the region of the bladder or kidneys, and *Nux* given every two or three hours.

INCONTINENCE OF URINE.

This may be occasioned by a weakness of the neck of the bladder, which is sometimes so great that a person is able to retain his water but a short time. The sitz-bath and electricity are valuable remedies. (See *Electricity.*)

Cantharides.—May be given six globules every night.

SEMINAL EMISSIONS.

This discharge frequently occurs in the young, just after reaching puberty, and is generally occasioned by irregular habits, and a morbid imagination.

The cultivation of a more healthy frame of mind, and, if remedies are required, the sitz-bath, and electricity, are all that will be required. (See *Electricity.*)

GONORRHEA—CLAP.

This disease consists of an inflammation of the urethra, (or passage from which the water is discharged), and only extends at first about an inch or two from the end of the penis. In from two to six days after an impure connection, a tingling or itching sensation is felt at the orifice of the urethra, especially when urinating. Soon the lips of the urethra become red and swollen, and the emission of urine is attended with burning, scalding pain. A discharge is now perceived, at first of a mucus character, but as the inflammation continues, becoming greenish or yellow. At night there may be painful erections of the penis.

Treatment.—During the inflammatory stage, characterized by painful swelling, and burning in passing water, *Aconite* and *Cantharides* should be given in alternation, three globules at a dose, three hours apart.

When the severity of the inflammation has subsided *Mercurius* may be given, six globules three times a day, followed by *Sulphur* at the same intervals, when the discharge becomes of a whitish character.

After the inflammatory symptoms have subsided, if the discharge should still prove obstinate, three drops of *Balsam Copaiva* may be given three times a day.

During the progress of the disease remain as quiet as possible, and avoid liquor and stimulating food. If the inflammation is severe the penis may be wrapped in cloths wrung out in cold water, and for the painful erections at night two drops of *Camphor* may be taken.

SYPHILIS.

Every discharge from the urethra may not be the result of an impure connection, neither is every sore upon the genitals syphilitic. The chancre usually presents itself at the end of the penis, in the form of a red itching pimple, from three to eight days after connection. If allowed to go on it gradually increases in size, until it becomes a large and deep ulcer. If the disease is not thoroughly exterminated from the system, often effects of the most serious character are the result, such as sores, eruptions, and a general breaking up of health.

Mercurius.—Taken morning and night, should commence the treatment, but the patient should lose no time in consulting a judicious physician. Avoid advertising quacks, for as a general thing they do much more harm than good.

CHAPTER X.

RHEUMATISM.

THIS extremely painful disease is very common in damp and changeable climates. Acute rheumatism is ushered in by a chilly sensation and a general sense of uneasiness. The joints are most liable to be affected, although the pain flies from one part of the body to the other. The pains are variable in character, dull, aching, or sharp, and aggravated by the slightest movement. There may be redness and swelling of the part affected, or these symptoms may be absent. In chronic rheumatism the pain is less severe, and is attended with no fever. In all forms of rheumatism the urine is acid and high-colored.

Treatment.—When there is much swelling or pain, cold or warm water may be applied, as is most agreeable to the patient. Six drops of *Arnica* may be mixed with three table-spoonfuls of water, and the swollen parts bathed with the mixture.

Aconite.—Should be given if much fever is present, quick pulse, heat, and dry skin. It may be alternated with *Belladonna*, *Rhus*, or *Bryonia.*

Belladonna.—Fever and pain in the head ; swelling,

with shining redness ; shooting pains, increased at night, and by a movement.

Bryonia.—Tearing pains increased by the slightest movement ; shivering, headache, and gastric symptoms.

Rhus.—Violent pains, worse at night, and in changeable weather, and relieved by motion.

Pulsatilla.—Pains, rapidly passing from one part to another, and relieved by exposing the part to the air.

Mercurius.—Pains increased by the warmth of the bed, by cold and damp air, and towards morning ; swelling of the parts ; perspiration, which, however, does not afford relief.

Nux-Vomica.—Tensive pains, particularly about the back, chest, and loins ; sensation of torpor, or numbness of the parts ; twitching of the muscles.

Dose.—In the early part of the disease, when considerable fever is present, it will often be advisable to alternate *Aconite* with some of the other remedies. Of the remedy selected give three globules every two, three or four hours, according to symptoms.

In *chronic* rheumatism lemon-juice will often be beneficial. *Sulphur* is also a valuable remedy, given morning and night. Great benefit also may be derived from the "*Galvanic Battery.*" (See *Electricity.*) For *Lumbago*, or pain in the back, *Nux*, *Bryonia*, *Rhus*, and *Pulsatilla*, are the prominent remedies ; fever, as directed above.

CHAPTER XI.

INJURIES FROM ACCIDENTS.

In our progress through the world, we are constantly liable to accidents and mechanical injuries, more or less severe. Occurring, sometimes, when it is impossible to obtain a physician or surgeon immediately, and when immediate action may not only prevent a vast amount of suffering, but even save life, every person should know what to do, until professional aid can be obtained. In all cases, when the injury is severe, a physician or surgeon should, of course, be obtained, as speedily as possible.

BURNS AND SCALDS.

In slight, superficial burns or scalds, the injured part may be held near the fire ; this, at first, may increase the pain, but in a short time produces entire relief. When the burn is not deep, *turpentine*, *alcohol*, *brandy*, or *rum*, warmed, may be applied, continuing to moisten the injured part until the pain is relieved.

A very excellent application, not only in deep and severe burns, but where they are more superficial, is *soap*. *Castile* or *white soap* should be scraped and made into a salve with tepid water, and this, spread on linen or muslin, applied over the whole injured part. This dressing may be changed, if necessary, once in twenty-four hours, being careful not to disturb the parts by washing. If blisters form puncture them with a needle, but do not expose the parts more than is necessary.

If the soap is too irritating, a very excellent and soothing liniment may be made by shaking thoroughly together equal parts of *sweet-oil* and *lime-water*. This liniment may be applied in the same way as the soap. Another very excellent application in extensive burns or scalds, is *wheat-flour*, dusted plentifully over the injured parts, keeping the parts constantly covered with the flour.

In scalds it is often necessary to cut the cloths, so as to remove them without producing serious injury. The garment should always be removed with the utmost care.

If much fever should be present, give *Aconite*, every two or three hours. If there should be trouble about the head, *Belladonna* may be given, and if there is much nervous excitement, *Rhus*.

SPRAINS.

A severe sprain is often more painful and tedious than a fracture or dislocation.

The injured part should be wrapped in cloths wet with cold water, or a mixture composed of one-fourth *Arnica* to three-fourths water. The same treatment may be pursued in bruises, mixing at the same time two drops of *Arnica* in a glass half-full of water, and giving a teaspoonful three times a day. When from a fall or blow the head or nervous system becomes affected, *Belladonna* may be alternated with the *Arnica* one, two, or three hours apart, as the symptoms indicate.

DISLOCATIONS.

Dislocations of the shoulder and elbow-joint are more common than any other. The appearance of the joint, compared with the one on the other side, together with the inability or great pain in moving the limb, point very clearly to the cause of the difficulty.

By a person possessed of a little mechanical skill, simple dislocations may be reduced with but little difficulty. Ascertain by careful examination the exact location of the old joint, and also of the end of the bone which has been forced from the socket. Move the opposite limb in different directions, watching carefully the action of the muscles. Then, with the thumb strongly pressed upon the end of the bone which has been forced from the socket, lift the injured limb carefully upwards, bringing it either forward or backward, all the time pressing with the thumb, making that the fulcrum, and the limb the lever. In this way a person, with a little care and thought, can often reduce a simple dislocation with but little trouble. In all cases a physician or surgeon should be obtained, if possible. When the dislocation is followed by much pain or swelling, cold water or *Arnica* may be applied in the same manner as directed for sprains.

FRACTURES.

A fracture can very readily be detected by a peculiar grating sound heard on moving the parts. This sound is occasioned by the ends of the fractured bones rubbing against each other. There is usually considerable pain, and more or less swelling.

The ends of the fractured bones should be brought carefully together, so, that when united, the limb shall be as nearly as possible as it was before it was broken. The limb should be kept perfectly still, all motion being prevented by means of splints placed by the sides of the limb, and the whole wound with a bandage. This, at first, should not be applied very tight for fear of swelling. If there is much swelling, cold water or *Arnica* should be applied, as directed for sprains.

WOUNDS.

Simple incised wounds are generally attended with no fever, and heal with but little trouble. Punctured, lacerated, or gun-shot wounds, on the contrary, are often attended with severe febrile disturbance, producing not unfrequently mortification and death. Incised wounds bleed freely, but lacerated or gun-shot wounds seldom cause much hemorrhage.

In all wounds the parts should be carefully washed, and all foreign substances removed. The hemorrhage may often be controlled by pressing the lips of the wound together with the finger, and the free application of cold water, or *Arnica* and water. If, however, one of the arteries is injured, which may be known by the bright red blood spouting out in jets at each pulsation of the heart, and the above measures do not check the hemorrhage, the current should be shut off by compressing the artery above the wound. To do this a piece of cork or pebble may be placed above the wound, directly on a line with the point from which the blood spouts. Over this, and around the entire limb a handkerchief may be tightly bound, introducing, if necessary, under the handkerchief a small stick, twisting it round. In this way the artery is compressed, and the hemorrhage immediately stopped. When the wound is in the lower part of the leg, the application should be made in the bend of the knee; when it is in the hand or forearm, in the bend of the elbow. The artery can now be readily tied with a thread. Cut from the *Arnica-plaster* (*Adhesive-plaster* will answer as well) long, narrow strips; moisten them, and, pressing the wound firmly together, place the strips across, so that they will extend some little distance over either side. If the wound is deep and gaping, it may be necessary to put in two or three stitches.

If much heat or swelling is present, the parts may be bathed with *Arnica* and water, or cold water. In deep, punctured wounds, it may be necessary, at first, to introduce lint, so that the wound may heal up from the bottom. This lint should be removed every day or two, and the parts washed with tepid water.

If considerable fever should set in, *Aconite* may be given once in two or three hours; if the parts are swollen and painful, *Belladonna* may be given at the same intervals.

STINGS OF INSECTS, AND BITES OF SERPENTS.

The bite of a poisonous serpent sometimes produces death in a few hours. The poison is speedily transmitted to every part of the system, and the remedy should be applied immediately. The wound should be exposed to *dry heat*, by means of a coal of fire, a hot iron, or even the stump of a cigar. The heated substance should be held as near the wound as possible without burning, and continued until a stretching, shivering sensation is experienced. When no fire can be obtained the poison may sometimes be sucked out with the mouth. *Oil*, *soap*, or *saliva* may be applied around the wound; a little *salt and water*, or *gun-powder*, may be taken into the mouth from time to time. If there are severe shooting pains, nausea, *Arsenicum* may be given every fifteen minutes.

The bite of spiders, mosquitoes, and other poisonous insects, and the sting of bees, may be relieved by bathing the parts with *Spirits of Ammonia* (*Spirits of Hartshorn*), or black garden mould may be placed over the swollen parts, renewing the application when the pain increases. For the sting of a bee in the mouth or eye, honey may be applied, smoke, tobacco smoke, or burning, brown sugar on coals will often drive off mosquitoes. The application of almost any alkali to the bite will produce relief.

CHAPTER XII.

APPARENT DEATH.

From Drowning.—Some persons on being precipitated into the water, stunned by the fall, or paralyzed by fear, sink like lead, and die without a struggle. Others struggle fearfully for life, rising to the surface of the water several times, and eagerly seizing hold of anything within their reach. Every time they come to the surface an attempt is made to obtain air, but usually water is introduced with it, which, exciting a cough, expels the little air introduced. The blood, from want of air, ceases to become arterialized, the action of the heart grows fainter and fainter, and, after the first struggle is over, the victim glides quietly, and almost with a sense of pleasure, into the arms of death. Death is not occasioned, as is sometimes supposed, by the admission of water into the lungs, for but very little, if any, is introduced, but simply from shutting off the necessary supply of air, by which the blood can become arterialized.

Often when persons are taken from the water apparently dead, life may be restored by well-directed and judicious efforts.

The mouth and nostrils should be cleansed, the wet clothes removed, and the body wiped dry and immediately covered with warm, dry clothes or blankets. If the weather is cold, this should be done on the spot, unless there is some dwelling close at hand.

These simple directions should always be observed, and all harsh usage or confusion avoided. Act energetically and with decision, but remember that confusion or failing to act right destroys the only chance for life.

In removing the body do not lift it by the shoulders and legs, so that the head falls backward and forward, but place it on a board or cart, in a recumbent posture, with the head and breast raised. On reaching the destination cover the body with warm, dry blankets, apply bottles of hot water to the feet and arm-pits. Keep the mouth and nostrils free, and the head and chest raised.

As soon as these preliminary steps have been taken, resort to artificial respiration. By means of a strip of cloth fit the tube of a common bellows accurately to one nostril, while the other is closed by the hand of an assistant, who, at the same time, closes the mouth.

Let another assistant with his right hand press backward, and draw gently downward toward the chest, the upper end of the wind-pipe, that prominence just below the chin, usually called *Adam's apple;* by doing this the passage to the stomach is stopped, while the wind-pipe is open for the free admission of air to the lungs. The left hand of the second assistant is to be spread lightly over the pit of the stomach, ready to compress the chest, and expel the air again, as soon as the lungs have been moderately filled; the first assistant unstopping the mouth and nostrils at the same time, to let the air escape. The same operation is to be repeated in a regular and steady manner, either until natural respiration begins, or until this and the other measures recommended, have been persisted in for three or four hours.

In the absence of the bellows, or until one can be procured, air can be blown into the lungs, by applying the mouth of the operator to that of the patient, and expelled in the manner directed above

While the process of artificial respiration is going on, others may be engaged in applying continued heat, such as dry, warm blankets, bottles of hot water, or hot bricks, and gentle friction with the hand.

A warm bath, not exceeding 100°, would also be of benefit. Slight shocks of electricity or galvanism passed through the diaphragm, or region of the heart, sometimes succeed when everything else fails.

The first signs of returning life are slight twitching of the muscles of respiration. When these signs are observed, the efforts should be increased, as the life of the patient can only be saved by continued exertion. As soon as the patient can swallow, a little brandy and water can, from time to time, be given. The return of life is often attended with the most intense pain. Even when the breathing has become calm, and the pulse regular, the patient should be closely watched for some hours.

Apparent Death from Hanging, Choking, or Smothering.—The treatment is precisely similar to that indicated in apparent death from drowning.

Apparent Death from Hunger.—Small injections of warm milk should be repeatedly given, and cloths, wet with warm brandy, placed on the stomach. As signs of returning life manifest themselves, warm milk may be given, a tea-spoonful at a time, to be followed, after a short interval, by a little beef-tea, or a few drops of wine, by degrees returning to a full diet.

Apparent Death from noxious Gases.—The presence of these gases, frequently found in wells, or where fomentation is going on, may be detected by lowering a candle ; if the candle goes out, the air will not support life ; while, if it burns brightly, there is no danger. In burning charcoal in an open room, the carbon of the coal, uniting with the oxygen of the air, forms carbonic acid gas, and unless the room is freely ventilated, the air soon becomes incapable of supporting life.

Remove the patient to the open air, dash cold water upon the face and chest, and employ artificial respiration as directed for drowning.

Apparent Death from Freezing.—The first symptoms of approaching danger is an irresistible drowsiness, which, if indulged, will soon glide into the sleep of death. When a person is found in this state, he should not be removed to a warm room, but to a place of shelter. If the body is stiff he should be covered several inches with snow, leaving the nostrils free. If snow cannot be obtained, place him in a bath of cold water. After the stiffness is removed by this treatment, gradually remove the clothes, cutting them off if necessary, and rub the body with snow, until it becomes red, or let it be placed in a room moderately warmed, covered with flannel, and briskly rubbed with the hands.

If still no signs of life show themselves, give every fifteen minutes an enema of *Camphor* and water.

As soon as the patient is able, let him swallow a little warm, black *coffee.* For the severe pains, which follow, give *Carbo-v.*, in alternation with *Arsenicum.* The patient should for some little time avoid the heat of the fire.

Apparent Death from Lightning.—Place the body in the open air, and dash cold water upon the face and chest. Should the body be cold, apply warmth or friction. Artificial respiration should be practiced as recommended for drowning.

A powder of *Nux-Vomica* may be placed on the tongue every fifteen or twenty minutes.

CHAPTER XIII.

POISONS AND THEIR ANTIDOTES.

In cases of poisoning, life itself may depend upon a prompt and vigorous treatment. Where poison has been taken into the stomach, it should be expelled as speedily as possible, by vomiting or the stomach-pump. If this cannot be done, some remedy should be administered, which will destroy the action of the poison.

Vomiting can generally be produced by introducing the finger into the throat, or by drinking freely of tepid water; also by placing snuff or mustard mixed with salt on the tongue. In some cases it will be necessary to give *Ipecac*, or *Tartar Emetic.*

Muriatic, Nitric, Oxalic, or *Sulphuric Acid.*—When poisoning occurs from these acids, if nothing else is at hand, drink freely of water, which will dilute the acid. Give immediately *Carbonate of Magnesia, Chalk, Old Mortar,* or even *Plaster*, scraped from the walls; or *soap-suds,* or *wood-ashes* mixed with water.

Arsenic.—Produce vomiting if possible, after which give *soap-suds*, or the *white of eggs.*

Corrosive Sublimate.—The *white of eggs* should be mixed with cold water, and given every two or three minutes, so long as the matter vomited contains a white opaque material, but when the substance vomited becomes transparent, no more should be given. If the *white of eggs* cannot be obtained, *soap and water* should be mixed with *wheat-flour*, and given plentifully.

Copper.—The *Acetate of Copper* is often formed in cooking-utensils, when they are not properly cleaned, in the form of *Verdigris.* Give freely of the *white of eggs,* or *sugar;* after vomiting has been produced give *Carbonate of Soda.*

Lead.—Poisoning from lead is common among painters, and where water is used which has been standing for some time in lead-pipes. (See *Lead Colic.*)

Poisonous effects are often produced by taking through mistake *Sugar of Lead.* Produce vomiting immediately, and then give dilute *Sulphuric Acid,* or *Epsom,* or *Glauber Salts.*

Tartar Emetic.—For the poisonous effects produced by *Tartar Emetic,* give strong *coffee, green tea,* or a decoction of *oak-bark.*

Tin.—Sour food allowed to remain in tin vessels, sometimes produces poisoning. Give the *white of eggs, sugar,* or *milk.*

Shellfish.—Sometimes produce vomiting. Encourage vomiting, and give *charcoal, sugar* and *water,* or strong *coffee.*

Animal Matter.—Rendered poisonous by putrefaction or disease. Give diluted *vinegar,* or *lemon-juice,* and afterwards strong *coffee.*

Nitre.—Saltpetre.—Produce vomiting by tepid water, afterwards give mucilaginous drinks, such as *gum-water*, or *flax-seed tea*.

Opium.—When this drug in the form of *Gum*, *Laudanum*, or *Morphine*, produces poisonous effects, vomiting should be produced as speedily as possible. As much *Tartar Emetic* as can be placed on a five cent piece, may be dissolved in a glass half-full of tepid water, and given a third every ten minutes, until vomiting takes place, giving in the intervals tepid water. When it is impossible to produce vomiting, it is necessary to use the stomach-pump. After some of the poison has been thrown from the stomach, give strong *coffee*, *vinegar*, or *lemon-juice*.

The strong desire to sleep should be prevented by walking the patient about, or dashing cold water into the face.

In poisoning from *Hyosciamus*, *Belladonna*, *Stramonium* (or *Stink-weed*), *Hemlock*, *Camphor*, *Strychnine*, *Lobelia* (or *Indian Tobacco*), and most of the other narcotics, the treatment is similar to that indicated for *Opium*.

Rhus.—Ivy.—The running or climbing *Ivy*, or, as it is sometimes called in the country, *Mercury*, will sometimes poison persons who come near it. It produces a perfect *Erysipelas*, with large blisters.

Bathing with *salt* and *water* will be of benefit. Take internally a cup of *coffee*, or three globules of *Belladonna*. The *Sumac* belongs to the same class of poison.

CHAPTER XIV.

ELECTRICITY.

Electricity and Magnetism perform an important part in every form of animal or vegetable life. Without them the earth would be a barren waste, and man could not exist. There would be no life-giving power in air or earth, no spiritual essence, developing in the world forms of beauty and fragrance, and peopling the earth with intelligent human beings. Deprive a plant of the action of these forces, generated in the earth and air, and it would die. Sever the nerve which transmits the nervous fluid from the brain to any organ, and that organ would cease to act. Flowing out from the brain, in whose secret chambers it is generated, the nervous fluid passes along the nerves of volition to every part of the body, communicating life and health. In the capillaries, that net-work which ramifies every part of the system, when the arteries and veins unite, the nerves of volition carrying the nervous fluid outward from the brain unite with the nerves of sensation, which carry impressions inward to the brain. Thus we have formed the complete circuit.

If then, from any of the numerous unhealthy influences to which we are exposed, this circuit in those minute capillaries is obstructed, pain is the result, and if the obstruction is complete, of course, in that part there is no action, and suppuration or disorganization of the parts ensues.

We can readily perceive then what an important agent electricity or magnetism must be in the cure of various forms of disease. The mildest form of magnetism is undoubtedly what is called animal magnetism, or the impression which one person may produce upon another through the action of the mind, and certain passes of the hands. When there is a high state of nervous excitement, or severe pain, this form of magnetism sometimes produces a very charming effect.

Almost every one has noticed the soothing effect produced in severe headache, or the restlessness of fever, by holding the hand on the head, or gently passing it over the forehead. When there is any seated pain, if muscular or nervous, passing the hand gently, in one direction, over the painful part, will often produce marked relief. In applying this form of magnetism, one hand may be placed on the head or the forehead, while the other holds a hand of the patient; or both hands may be pressed on the head, or passes may be made downward, or the hand passed gently in one direction over the painful part. If the impression is too strong it will be only necessary to reverse the passes.

Next to Animal Magnetism we may notice the Electro-Magnetic or Electro-Galvanic Battery. In many forms of disease, the Battery, properly constructed and applied, is a powerful remedial agent. In paralysis, neuralgia, chronic rheumatism, abcesses, spinal difficulties, and weakness or inaction of any organ, it may be used with decided benefit. The battery, however, should be properly constructed, and the power so nicely adjusted, that the current will be scarcely perceptible, and can be applied with safety to the most delicate and vital organ, or increased, so as to produce violent muscular contraction

Another important point is to have the shocks all in one direction, and the *positive* and *negative* pole always remain *positive* and *negative.* In most of the batteries the poles constantly change, so that there can be no continued current along the nerves, breaking down obstructions, and restoring a natural nervous circulation.*

In applying the battery for the first time, the patient can take hold of one pole, and the operator of the other, while with the other hand he manipulates about the diseased part of the patient. In this way the shocks may be given with great benefit and safety.

Another very excellent way is to attach to one or both of the poles a moist sponge. If one pole is held in the hand of the patient, let the moist sponge of the other be passed along the diseased part. When there is great spinal weakness, or general inaction of the system, it can be passed down the spine. Or the operator, taking hold of the non-conducting

* One of the best Batteries now in use, combining in a very happy manner these principles, is one recently invented by Dr. Carpenter. It is not expensive and is very compact in its form.

portions of the poles, can hold the sponges on either side of the diseased part. In cases of muscular contraction, it may be necessary to apply the poles without the sponges, being careful to send the shocks along the course of the nerves.

In applying the battery to any delicate or vital organ, it should be applied with great care, for if the shocks are too strong, serious consequences, and, perhaps, even death may be the result.

THE END.

INDEX.

CARPENTER'S
MAGNETO-MEDICAL BATTERY.

A New Machine for Medical purposes, arranged without Acids.

By Dr. C. CARPENTER, Jr.

ELECTRICITY, in some form or other, plays an important part in all animal and vegetable life. In the human frame its subtle influence is diffused throughout the whole system ; disturb its equilibrium or cut it off from any portion of the system, and pain and disease is the result.

This powerful agent, properly applied, through a carefully prepared Magneto-Electric Battery, is of immense importance in the treatment of diseases, and will render the cure of many of those painful maladies which have heretofore bid defiance to human skill, simple and easy. All of those troubles characterized by a general inaction of the system, or of particular organs,are speedily relieved by means of electricity. In the treatment of female diseases, in neuralgia, paralysis, rheumatism, deafness, weakness of sight, and partial blindness, the magnetic or galvanic battery is regarded by the medical profession as one of the most powerful remedial agents in their possession. The electric current breaks down the obstructions of disease, and stimulates with new life parts which were before debilitated and almost inactive.

Recently, scientific research has brought to light a NEW FACT, which must be hailed with delight by thousands, whose days and nights are now filled with suffering. This fact is the power of the Magneto-Electric Battery of freeing the system from those mineral substances such as MERCURY and LEAD, which, either in the form of medicine or by being constantly exposed to their influence in many of the employments of life, enter the system, producing fearful diseases, which have heretofore dragged the poor victim to an early grave. By the *Magneto-Electric Battery* the system may be easily freed from these substances in a similar way that the electrotyper precipitates upon the article intended to be elec-typed, the silver, gold or copper. By applying the poles of the battery with the proper solution, the precipitate always takes place on the substance in contact. So in the human frame; by placing the patient in a bath, expressly and carefully prepared, and applying the battery, the mineral is forced out of the system and precipitated on the sides of the bath. To do this however, the *battery* must be so constructed that the current is always in its full strength, in *one direction*, and the positive and negative poles always remain the same. THIS FEATURE is peculiar to *Dr. Carpenter's* battery, and renders it infinitely superior, as a remedial agent, to any other in use.

Another important feature in this battery is the much improved plan for increasing the rapidity of the shocks, so that a continuous and pleasant current can be produced. The absence of acids, and the ease with which the instrument can be graduated, so that it can be applied with perfect safety to the most delicate organ, or increased in continuous power to produce violent muscular contraction, very greatly enhances its value. *The scale* by which the power can be measured, the compact form of the instrument, added to its other most important improvements, must introduce it to popular favor, more especially as it is *not* liable to lose its power or to get out of order.

The *attention* of the *medical profession*, as well as the public, is most earnestly solicited to the peculiarities and improvements of this instrument.

Twelve dollars is the price for a Machine adapted for general use, with the addition of extra apparatus for physicians, according to its extent.

It may be had of OTIS CLAPP, Beacon street, Boston, of WILLIAM RADDE, New York, and of dealers in Chemical and Electrical Instruments generally; also, of regular Druggists and Apothecaries, both of the *Allopathic* and *Homœopathic* Schools of Medicine.